My Journey with Leukemia

The Power of Family, Faith, and Humor

Jennifer Slaughter Venegas

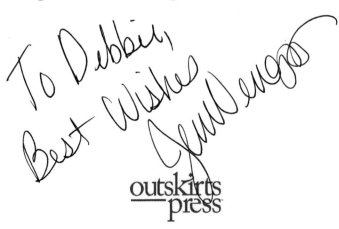

To Debbie,
Best Wishes
Jen Venegas

outskirts
press

Acknowledgments

As I read though the book again, I praised and thanked a lot of people along my journey. That being said, I feel it's necessary to recognize the people who saved my life and gave me the strength to persevere and continue my search for normal.

To GOD. My healer, my strength, my heart, my life. Who was with me putting things in place and placing people in my life for my good YEARS before my diagnosis. Who sat with me, prayed with me, listened to me, carried me, and gave me hope. Who cried for me. And who guides me to this day.

Rebecca Slaughter. My savior. The reason I am still here today. Without your lifesaving stem cells, I literally would not be here now. I really don't have the words to express how sincerely thankful I am for you in my life. You endured the agonizingly painful process in preparation of the stem cell harvest without question. You know me better than I know myself. We are forever connected and I thank God for you.

To Joe and John. I can't imagine what you went through. I wasn't on your side of the bed. I don't know what it was like to see me in such pain, fighting for my life, enduring unbelievable torture, and not being able to do anything. You took it one day at a time and did your best to wake up every day and continue to live your lives the best you could. John, I never wanted you to be a kid whose mom had cancer. You'll have that "title" and experience for the rest of your life, and I'm so sorry. But you never acted like a victim and you managed the unthinkable when faced with the reality you might lose your mom. You were forced to grow up WAY too fast, and you did it mostly on your own. You always knew what to say to make me smile and you gave me purpose to survive.

To my husband Joe. I don't have the words. I can't possibly ever imagine what this has been like for you, and yet you're still here with me. You always seem to know what to say to calm me down, help me breathe, and keep me in line. You were thrown into your own hell but survived it and we emerged, still together, on the other side. I owe everything to you. You were forced into the unthinkable role of being everything to both John and me. A rock. Mom, dad, husband, bill payer, worrier, worker, cleaner, single provider, and on and on. In a much different way, I believe you survived as much hell and agony as I did and entirely alone. You had John, and my family took great care of me so you could focus on being the bread winner and be all for John, but that had to feel impossible every day. Yet, you worked overtime, went to John's games, was the ultimate parent, and managed to find the strength to overcome. I also never wanted you to be the husband whose wife had cancer, and I know it's not my fault, but I'm so sorry you had to, and still have to live this unthinkable reality and new normal with me. I love you so much.

To my Slaughter family: Mom, Dad, Stephanie, Rebecca and Ryan. As in true Slaughter form, you circled the wagons from the moment I was diagnosed and experienced your own new normal as I went through the treatment and recovery process. You took care of me so completely and with such amazing grace. You fought for me and my family. You came to my room at all hours of the day, before the sun rose, in the middle of the night, when I was in crippling pain, when I was incoherent. I am truly blessed to have you in my life and know I couldn't have made it through that hell without your love, support, prayers, and doing the things I didn't know you were doing behind the scenes. Thank you from the bottom of my heart.

To the Amazing Dr. Hyde, who literally saved my life overnight. If he hadn't been there that first night, I'm certain I would not have made it through the night. He's initial bedside manner was very direct, scientific, and unattached, but his absolute dedication to the practice of medicine and specialty of Oncology was unparalleled. He is brilliant, and I am honored to say he always had my back and made true every promise he made. My soul was in his hands and he cherished, nurtured, and saved it.

To the nurses, who are the true heroes. They knew just as much if not more than the doctors AND with grace, patience, love, and kindness. They did everything in their power to maintain my dignity and understood, to the best of their ability, the torture they were delivering, knowing it was the only way to save my life. I still see them from time to time and they have become friends.

To Dr. Gregory (SCT) and Dr. Eisenstein (Oncology) who have been fabulous throughout all this. They listened to my concerns, treated me with respect, and helped me see there can be a tomorrow. They also valued me as an individual and addressed each and every concern with the newest possible treatments. I was a willing Guinea Pig for nearly everything they tried, knowing they were doing the best they could with my insanity.

To Margaret, my rock. I was at your home in Houston when I started to recognize, really feel, like something was wrong. I was light headed and dizzy and we both just thought it was the altitude or travel sickness. Now we both know you were witnessing the beginning of my death. You were the first person I called that night I was diagnosed and my go-to person throughout my ordeal. You were there when I was crying and scared. You were there in the middle of the night when I needed to hear a voice. You created my Facebook page and kept me sane. You updated my CaringBridge when I couldn't, and gave me a safe place in my mind. I knew I could count on you for anything, and still wear that amazing comfy robe. That was incredibly soothing to me and a staple in all my hospital visits. I still feel safe when I wear it and smile when I think of you.

To my Angel Team. EVERYONE who prayed for me, supported my family, sent positive thoughts, made meals or gave rides, gave me pedicures and massages, sent cards, followed my CaringBridge and Facebooks accounts, supported me through your thoughts and words, asked how I was doing, and stuck with me through thick and thin. Those who planned the benefit event and made sure we could survive financially. It was in your strength that I relied on and knew it would always be there.

To the facilities that participated in my recovery: Rock Creek Medical Center and Kaiser Permanente, Presbyterian/St. Luke's Hospital, Colorado Blood Cancer Institute,

To the organizations that are committed to the patients and their caregivers. Who give us support, hope, and information. BMTInfonet.org, Immerman Angels, The

Leukemia and Lymphoma Society, The Cancer Society, Domus Pacis, and on and on. I named the ones I was particularly involved with.

And to www.Caringbridge.com who made this book possible. It was because of their website I was able to communicate with family and friends and gave me a platform to just write. It was instrumental to my healing and recovery for so many reasons. I vented. I explained. I praised. I asked for help. I spewed. I processed and reflected and prayed. I just wrote. And other people could respond, which was lifesaving to me. Knowing I truly wasn't alone in my lonely hospital room, in my home, in my travels, was critical to my mental and physical health. The encouraging thoughts gave me hope and made me believe I could do it because I wasn't alone. And gave me strength through their thoughts and prayers and encouraging words that I never would have had alone. If it wasn't for the CaringBridge website, I truly believe I'd be much worse than I am and can't thank them enough. Please consider donating to the website as it can only continue through the donations from others. Thank you to those of you whom already did.

Table of Contents

Prologue

Six months before I heard the words I didn't understand, I started noticing things change in my body I couldn't explain or put together. As a woman, you just know when things aren't right but can't explain how, and if you tried to tell a doctor, they'd just give you a med or single diagnosis (infection) and not put it all together. I was getting unexplained and random fist sized bruises on my legs, torso, and arms. I had one infection after another: bladder, yeast, colds. My stomach was always upset. I felt severely hungover every day, without having had a single drop of alcohol the night before. I had lost my mental sharpness and was confused all the time. My gums were bleeding for no reason and the dentist though it was gum disease. I started having periods after nearly 5 years of not having them. I was getting headaches. I noticed I didn't have any energy and couldn't even walk up a flight of stairs. I'd get half-way up and have to pause to catch my breath, and then again when I reached the top. Two months before I was diagnosed, I visited a dear friend in Texas and felt lightheaded or dizzy all the time. We explained it off as altitude or travel sickness. I had plenty of energy and even assembled a bed and managed to fix a tech issue with her TV's. Nothing's wrong here, right?

In December, one month from my new life, I decided enough was enough and lived a "clean life". No alcohol, a healthy diet, sleep/rest. And yet things just got worse. I dreaded the worst. A heart issue. Lung disease. Tumor somewhere. So the first day back to work I told my supervisor of my concerns (I almost fainted twice during the staff development), that I wanted to go to the doctor, and they sent me on my way with a great deal of worry.

I went to my doctor and she thought I was having heart issues. But the EKG came up normal. Then it was to imaging to scan my lungs. Also normal. As a last resort, they took some blood, left me in the treatment room to get my flu shot, and gave me a script for anxiety and anxiety attacks. Yep, anxiety attacks. I KNEW it wasn't anxiety attacks, but who was I to question their professional opinion?

Until the doctor came back and said the blood tests had some abnormalities and I was very anemic. She recommended I get to the ER ASAP. Ok. Nothing to worry about. A little Iron and I'll be fine.

Nope. I got to the ER and my doctor had already sent them my test results. I didn't know it then, but as I look back, they were worried. They rushed me back to a room, and immediately took me in for an MRI. I called my sister and husband and told them I was in the ER, thought it was anemia and no big deal, but the staff told me to get people there to help me.

They asked me all kinds of questions and were worried because I was bleeding out somewhere. I had no red blood cells. At this point though, I was dying. My sister understood and noticed I was literally turning grey. My life was leaving me. Joe got there and I felt like all would be ok, but honestly, I was delirious.

Then someone (Dr. Hyde) came in and said, "Well, you've got it". I remember that, but I didn't know what "it" was. Then he told us I had a 30 day stay in the hospital. My first thought was, "What about work? That can't be possible. I have to work tomorrow. What do I need to do to get out of here?"

The rest becomes weird. They were looking for a room to admit me. My thoughts, "Cool. Whatever." No idea of the danger I'm in. I got a room and called Mom and told her I had Leukemia. I still didn't know what that meant, but I kinda knew I was in trouble.

I got up to my room, and they already had a bag of blood waiting for me. I was so out of it though, I felt like I was checking into a hotel or something. And I'm still wondering what I'm going to do about work. Denial.

Even the next day, and 2 bags of blood later, I had no idea what was going on. They were talking in a different language using words like neutropenia, chemo, stem cell transplant, bone marrow biopsy, transfusions, PICC line. I was still so sick though none of it really registered. I was going through the motions and would be for the next 6 months. This is the beginning of my story.

Chapter 1

The Journey Begins

My Story
January 8, 2014

Hey Everyone,
I have some news to share with you and unfortunately, it is not the kind of news you want to hear. As you know, I am one to say it like it is and get to the point, so here it goes:

After feeling weak and sick for a few weeks, I went to the doctor this past Monday. After a blood test, which led to a bone marrow biopsy, I was diagnosed with Acute Lymphocytic Leukemia. Yep. Not great news. More tests are being run to determine the exact strain and hence the exact course of treatment. However, for now I will be receiving an aggressive regimen of chemotherapy which we hope will eradicate the cancer cells. I may or may not be looking at a bone marrow transplant in the future. Again, this will depend on further test results coupled with my system's reaction to the chemotherapy.

I will be in the hospital for around a month as we work through this. I would love to not only hear from you but would like for you to receive updates as they become available. At this time, I cannot receive visitors or flowers, unfortunately, because I must be in complete isolation free from all germs but welcome your love and support. Your thoughts and prayers are so important to me and I want to hear from you as I travel through this difficult time. As any mother would, my biggest concern is helping Joe and John cope with this as well. Please keep Joe and John in your thoughts. As with any other household, you are never prepared for an extended absence of the "mother of the house". You can help us in many ways. Gift cards (restaurants, Walmart, movies, etc.), meals, gifts/cards, and time (taking the boys to a movie or dinner, etc.).

Because my job will be to focus on my health and may not have the time and energy, we (actually my dear friend Margaret) created a page on Caringbridge.com called "Jennifer Venegas" to communicate my status and receive notes from you. She (Margaret) also set up a page on Facebook called Team Jennifer Venegas. PLEASE Feel free to join either of these sites (or both) and share them with others I may have missed through FB and email. We will be posting updates on this site frequently, so you can check whenever you'd like to see what's happening as I make this journey to health and wholeness. Likewise, you can leave me messages!
Things you can do to help...

Use the websites to post uplifting thoughts or stories, post pictures, make donations, sign the guestbook, etc. I'll be hungry for outside exposure and news!
Stay in contact with Joe...he needs support
Stay in contact with John...text, call, etc.
Meals for Joe and John.
Help with motherly chores (house cleaning, events with John, etc.)
Prayers and positive thoughts.
Please keep my family and me in your prayers and keep positive thoughts. I'm a fighter and plan to beat this. With your love and support I know I can.

Love, Jenn

Building Up to Tear Down
January 9, 2014

The first thing they did when I got here 3 days ago was hook me up to blood transfusions to build up my system to a point where they aren't afraid I'll die. When I came in 3 days ago, my blood levels were so low I was literally bleeding out and turning grey. They weren't sure I would make it through the night. Thank God I did, but I still had no idea what I was up against. I still don't know what Leukemia is. Is that cancer? A disease? Dr. Hyde has been terrific in trying to fill us in on the details, but honestly all I know is I'm still too sick to survive chemo, which is what is next. I guess that means I have cancer. But what does that mean? My brain hurts from thinking about it. The nurses tell me my numbers, but I have no idea what they mean. I wake up and wait to see what the plan is and have no choice but to go with the plan. As soon as my levels are high enough, they'll start destroying them with chemo and so it begins. The only word I have is surreal.

The battle begins - with a hiccup
Jan 10, 2014

Started the chemo prep today. Although I had an allergic reaction to one of the meds, the Dr. (Hyde...ha ha) was all over it. He had a plan B all ready to go and we're still going. I'm so ready for this fight. It's like the suspense of fighting it is worse than what it is. I know I've got a huge fight, but the doctor is so darn positive it's contagious. We are a team and he's got me in his hands.

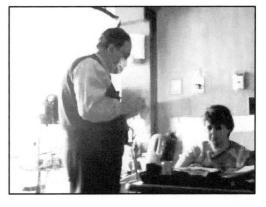

I'm also taking every little piece of news as a small miracle. I know I am already fighting this thing. My white blood cell count (the enemy) has dropped and I'm out of that danger for now. All the tests (CT, PET, lung X-ray, EKG, ultrasound, blood work) indicate the cancer is confined to just the lymph (the "water" that travels with the blood) ...WHICH IS EXCELLENT NEWS!! Each one of those test results created a celebration and prayer of blessing and praise. I have an amazing support team that is so far reaching I can't believe it. People are talking about having stem cell drives. My tears are often tears of happiness and humility and relief. In tough times you really discover who the people are that have your back, and I am truly blessed. More than I'll EVER know.

Funny
Jan 11, 2014

Yesterday I had to get a PET scan which injects radioactive sugar water that attaches to cancer cells and shows up on a CAT scan. They look for masses and tumors. The good news is that the test came back negative! Yee haw! The funny... The PET scanner is in a building 100 yards from the hospital. I had to be transported via wheelchair and ambulance, about a 30 second drive, and back for the test. Laughable!!! As I returned to the hospital, the automatic doors wouldn't open. The EMT was livid. After about 20 seconds the doors opened, and we were assaulted by a nurse and the whole security staff, you know, the rent-a-cops. They were looking for someone that tripped the alarm thus locking the door. No one but us. The staff was baffled...until they asked who I was and where I was coming from. Apparently, the radioactive material they injected in me set off the alarm!!! And no... I checked. I didn't glow in the dark!

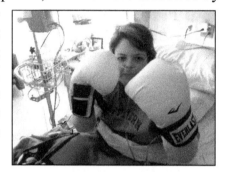

Julie - Hahaha. That is funny. The funniest is that you checked to if you were glowing. Sounds like a bit of good news. Love that!
Rex - You've been GLOWING since I 1st saw you arrive here 42 years ago honey! LOL Keep on glowing babe...I LOVE IT!!!!!

Update
Margaret - Jan 12, 2014

Hello, all! *It's Margaret, Jenn's friend. I talk/text with Jenn every day several times and want to add a few updates. Jenn began chemotherapy yesterday, with continuation today. Although there were a few hiccups yesterday, she is doing great today and is on a chemo drip that is zapping that stupid "Raider" which is her name for the you know what. She has had moments of anxiety and being scared (jeez...who wouldn't?) but is remaining strong and confident that she will have a full recovery. Right now, she is VERY concerned about her beloved Broncos, but that is in Peyton Manning's hands. :-)*

I will continue to keep you all updated. I look forward to the day when my post will be my last, when it will simply say, "CURED." Keep those positive thoughts and prayers headed Jenn's way!

<u>Jeana</u> - Thank you for your updates and for being such a great support to Jenn. Looking forward to that final post you mention.

Broncos!
Jan 12, 2014

Whew! I made it through another treatment without any negative reactions. And the Broncos pulled off another win. I couldn't be happier. It was a good day. Thank you everyone for the positive and motivating thoughts! Your support is so important to my recovery and I appreciate you all so much. Love!!

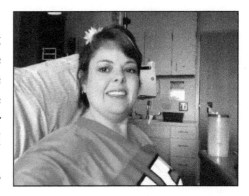

<u>Rex</u> - Great day...both Jennifer & the Broncos won!!!!! I'm happy, happy, happy! :-)

Update
Margaret - Jan 13, 2014

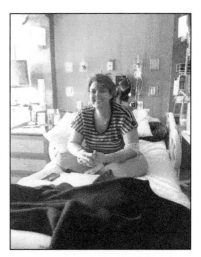

Hi, everyone. Jenn is feeling relatively great still and seems to be tolerating the chemo well! She received more chemo and platelets this morning and a lumbar tap to explore and administer a precautionary dose of chemo to the spinal fluid. More chemo tonight with a stronger dose and then a huge dose on Wednesday. Hopefully she will be able to keep up the tolerance level. What she really wants is a beer and I don't blame her! I especially felt bad that she could not partake in her favorite beverage last night when the Broncos kicked butt! More later!

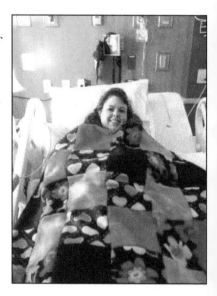

Stephanie - Busy day today. Chemo this morning, a lumbar puncture and test, more aggressive round of chemo this evening. Lots going on. Great day for extra prayer and encouragement. A lot more anxiety and nerves today. It can be tricky to lay in bed and forfeit control, even though she is surrounded by very capable hands. Thanks for your support!

** Don't you LOVE my blanket? Mom made a blanket for each new hospital visit. The special blankets were essential for my comfort. I still have them all and treasure them! **

Test results
Jan 14, 2014

The lumbar tap yesterday was clear and normal. No headaches or reactions. Today is the last day of the second round of treatments with some transfusions to build me back up. It's been a great day emotionally, spiritually, and physically. Tomorrow is the last round of chemo with a super-duper 24-hour dose that should really put the cancer on the run. Show it who's boss. I'm feeling strong, blessed, and supported.

Gina - Jenn, you are an inspiration! Prayers are coming your way for sure! Good luck tomorrow.
Rex - You're kicking ass honey! One more day of chemo & I pray you'll be on 3rd base heading for home plate...you're in the red zone & ready for a TD!!!!! Makes me excited & happy, happy, happy for you babe! I have great faith you will get thru this ordeal & move on w/ your blessed life. Love ya, lots, DAD ;-)

Tough night
Jan 15, 2014

I had a tough night last night, buzzers, bad dreams, and such. But a new team of nurses, a shower, a prayer, and mom put me back in line. Also a few laps around the floor took the Dr.'s fears away from my low heart rate. The Chardonnay colored chemo was a definite pick me up. My bright pink blanket and robe are also a hit. My nurse and life saver (Eric) wondered where the battery pack was for the robe. Lol. All is well!

While I'm on the Eric subject, he is my angel. He was here the first day I was here, and the chaos set in. My family was here, we didn't know anything about Leukemia, nurses were in and out, we hadn't figured out the routine, or how to order food, or where my family could rest or eat or use the bathroom. It was a hot mess. And Eric noticed my confusion and ho overwhelmed I was. He took me aside and gently talked to me about what to expect and ways to cope. And the best advice he gave me was to find the positive every day. No matter how bad the day is, find something to be grateful for and write it down. And you know what? It works. The minute I took a minute to seek what is positive, I immediately calm down and stopped thinking about me and my situation. I started seeing how everything could be worse. That other people have their own things too. And my worst day is better than someone's best day. It's true. I had running water and a bathroom to myself. I was in a top-notch hospital with a solid roof and no bombs going off around me. I had family and friends. The sun came up and I'm still here. I had my arms and legs and was otherwise healthy…you know, other than the cancer. My family had a warm place to live and cars to drive, and food on the table. What did I have to worry about?

Rex - Love it that u r feeling better today after a very difficult night. Between Dr. Hyde, Eric & your mother around it must've lifted your spirits a little bit! ;-)
Ryan - You're a warrior. I love you!
Tammy - I am thinking of you. Which hospital are you in? Once upon a time I was a bone marrow transplant nurse at Presbyterian/ St Luke's. Great group of doctors and nurses everywhere who will give you their best every day!
Julie - I love that bright blanket, matches your personality. Keep fighting girl!
Lana - My heart and prayers are with you Jen ♡
Dana, sends her love and she was very upset when she heard that you were not feeling good 😍

Amy - Jennifer, you don't know me but your sister, Steph, shared your story. You're. my hero. your strength and faith are an inspiration. I'll be praying, you keep fighting.

Outpouring
Jan 16, 2014

I am so overwhelmed by the outpouring of love, attention, faith, thoughts, prayers, and actions from you all. It's one thing to feel it for myself, but the way you have enmeshed and supported my sisters, brother, parents, husband and son in the same ways are as equally remarkable. I have a big ol' care team that just keeps growing. I can't thank you enough!!

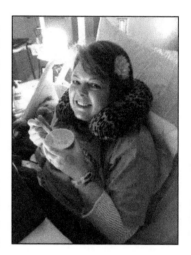

I did not ask for this, do not want to be anyone's hero, or inspiration, strength, or motivation, but your prayers and words and support make me see it's not my fight alone to face. This is, and will be a team effort and I can't imagine a single moment of it without any of you on my side.

I... AM...BLESSED!!!!

Laura - Jenn, I haven't met you before, but I work with Steph every morning in her classroom. Just wanted you to know that I've been praying for you before I even knew there was anything going on with you, just knew Steph was really upset but she couldn't talk about it yet. Just knew God knew what was wrong and would cover it in prayer. Since then prayers have been coming your way for healing, strength, comfort and peace for you; strength, comfort and peace for all of your family members; wisdom for your doctors and just that all of you would feel God's loving arms wrapped around you, giving you His peace that surpasses all understanding. You also have the prayers of the women in my bible study and the prayers of the prayer team at Boulder Valley Christian Church! Keep up the good fight and find your strength in Him!

Rex - Jennifer - Here I come...like it or not! LOL ;-) DAD
Joan - You must feel like you are in a love cocoon. Your team is growing, and we are united in prayers (and throw in some orange also) for you. I will be thinking of you today.

Dad
Jan 17, 2014

I can't tell you how special the days have been having you in my room to chat, and nap, and watch TV and just connect with you. This is really hard, but daddies make it all better. After you left I started that new chemo pill and it's been a little bummer. I'm sleeping though and with an amazing team and good hands. They've got my back here while you have it in my heart.

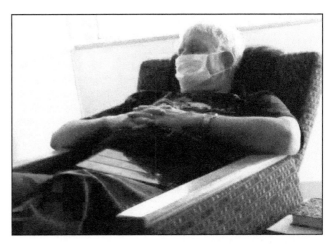

Rex - Aaaaaw ... You make my heart soar like an eagle ;-) What a special person you are. I'm couldn't be any PROUDER of what you have become honey! I love being your DAD now & forever honey ;-)
Karen - The Illinois Walkers send our love. One of my favorite quotes: "For I can do everything through Christ, who gives me strength". Praying for strength and comfort for you and the entire family. Love you

Birthday?

Jan 18, 2014

It seems absolutely ridiculous to be celebrating a birthday in here. Weird. Abnormal. I'm in a hospital room, have been for almost 2 weeks, and most of all of this has been foggy at best. What do you do when you're in the hospital on your birthday? Well, the nurses were terrific! They brought me balloons and sang happy birthday. And my family visited and texted and called. It's still surreal though.

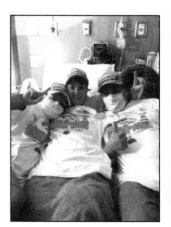

And when you have your birthday while fighting a killer and uncertainty is the only future you have, now what? Will I see another birthday? How many will I have? It's unthinkable, really. Another year? More? Less? All I have is today. So, I'm going to take a shower and put on clean clothes and see what my stomach can handle. And be happy I made it this far.

Champs!

Jan 19, 2014

And my boys brought me a Championship shirt and hat even though I wasn't able to go. I've never felt more loved!

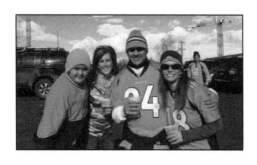

Side Effects Stink
Jan 20, 2014

So, I've been here in the hospital for 2 weeks now. Not in a million years did I ever see this coming when I walked into the ER 2 weeks ago today for some blood tests. I haven't been home since. I haven't seen my dog, I haven't slept in my bed, and I haven't had a minute of normal since. The first week was testing and receiving chemo. Now the chemo is doing its job and essentially killing everything good, and bad, so my body can do a re-boot and start downloading and rebuilding the healthy again. And just when I think a "round" is over, I get another "booster" dose of chemo. Like today; I'll be going in for another Lumbar Tap and chemo shot. I feel like crap. As much 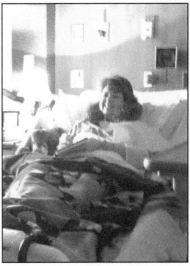 as I want to move around, the more I move, the more I hurt something. The headaches are the worst.

I told Dr. Hyde he can only come in my room if he has good news from now on. The first time I said this, he responded without losing a beat, *"Well you're not pregnant"*. He's a terrific guy and is really working with me on the best treatment for my very rare and unique type of Leukemia. Today's comment was that he expects me to start feeling better in the next few days (at least there's a goal). He also said my CT (MRI) and other follow up tests are clear or normal. This is good news indeed!

More to come...

Ryan - Clear and normal is terrific. I hope the headaches subside. I know how bad that must be. Love you!
Julie - That's great news from Dr. H!
Eldon - When the going gets tough, the tough get going. From everything I've read you are as tough as they come. From the Arnold family to the Slaughter family, especially you Jennifer, our prayers are with you. Hang in there.
Tammy - Thinking of you!
Rex - We'll celebrate even the small victories like being told you will feel better in a few days! I love the Dr.'s good news & I am very proud of the dignity & strength

of character you have shown during these horrible & painful chemo treatments!
Jenn you're the best of the best! Love ya always, DAD
Kathy - Your post about Dr. Hyde's comment made me LOL, really! What would we
do in life without humor? Keep it up and know we are rooting for you all the way
from Illinois!

Ups and Downs
Jan 21, 2014

I must say, I was totally unprepared for this. Duh, I guess. And I have been fortunate enough to never have experienced a cancer diagnosis from a friend or family member that required Chemotherapy. My father is a survivor and if I'm anything like him at all, which I am, I'm going to be fine.

They're still trying to find the right combinations of medications to give me. And each medication also then required pre-meds for the side-effects. And sometimes counteract those as well. I'm allergic to the only pain pill that relieves the headache pain, so I have to take a Benadryl with it. Unbelievable. With all this chemo and medications, I wonder how much of me will still be here in the end. Hopefully, just the good parts!

They are going to do an ECHO this afternoon, so we'll see how that goes. Hopefully their concerns about my heart are unfounded and just a side effect of the meds. Wish me luck!

Rex - Mom said spinal tap was ok & you're eating now & the headache is better...TERRIFIC! Get a nice massage & rest if u can today. See ya tomorrow like it or not babe! Better hide your Elway autographed photo...LOL

Too much info?
Jan 23, 2014

Apparently one of the side effects of all this is an occasional night with no sleep. Thought I'd take the sleepless time and update the tests I've had and the results. In the beginning, all the tests were done for diagnosis, ruling in/out, and baseline purposes. From here on out the tests will be to determine change.

EVERY CLEAR OR NORMAL RESULT WAS FOLLOWED BY A CELEBRATION!!!

Chest x-ray - Clear.

CT Scan of brain - Clear.

MRI of brain - Clear. However, if they ever want another one of those on me again, they will have to keep it a secret and sedate me - put me under totally - for that to happen. If you've ever had your head in a tin bucket with 30 kindergarteners banging on it with every conceivable implement imaginable (rocks, sticks of varying thickness and tone and the instructions "be creative - express yourself", no rhyme or rhythm, and humming through kazoos) WHILE you're experiencing the worst hangover headache and nausea, then you have a shadow of how that felt to me.

Blood tests - Revealed anemia and other blood count abnormalities, specifically the ALL diagnosis. Many of these tests were sent to cancer centers throughout the country for evaluation. The blood tests are daily and will continue.

Bone Marrow and Tissue Biopsy - Yes, it hurt like hell. The cells they pulled from my hip were also sent to cancer centers around the country for evaluation. I'll probably need at least one more, and depending on the success of the chemo, another one may be needed for a blood marrow transplant.

Lumbar Tap (good ole' spinal tap - just sounds nicer) - To extract brain and spinal cells and to administer a chemo shot. So far, the results of the tests are clear, and the injections are for preventative purposes. Another 4-6 of these will be necessary before it's all said and done. And no, it doesn't hurt (like an epidural).

Ultrasound - Kidneys, Liver, Bladder, Gall Bladder, Appendix, Intestine, Stomach, and any other organ in my abdomen. All clear.

EKG (heart) - Thankfully I was born with dad's cardiopulmonary system and was blessed with a low heart rate and low blood pressure. Unfortunately, that doesn't work to my favor in this case. I've been monitored closely, and I'm just fine.

ECHO Cardiogram - A very detailed, live action ultrasound of my heart and by far the most beautiful thing I've ever seen in my life, and something I would never have the words to truly express my awe. I saw and heard my heart beating. It was miraculous. Beautiful. And results came back clear. (Except for some silly little abnormal heart something or another that has nothing to do with this, has no bearing on this, and will never be mentioned again for as long as I live).

PET Scan - A radioactive, full body CT scan. Came back normal. I wrote a journal entry on this funny story several days ago.

Well, that's about it for now and I think I'm up to date on all previous tests. Keep moving forward and fighting whatever comes at me.

Ryan - Thanks for this update. I didn't sleep last night either. I loved your explanation of the MRI, u had me giggling.

Rex - It sounds pretty good to me! Makes me happy & less anxious than I was a couple of weeks ago...I pray that your bod will continue to get stronger & kick this leukemia in the ass!!!!! Love ya always & forever. BTW - I had one of those MRI tests before my cancer surgery a few years ago & nearly lost mind...that is what's left of it! Strapped my arms & head down & it took (as I recall) 2 or 3 days (lol) to go through this claustrophobic nightmare of grief! NOT FUN!!!!! Hope neither of us have to ever endure that torture machine ever again. It ranks 2nd to the "SCREAMING EAGLE " @ Six Flags in Missouri - REMEMBER? I got bruises on my arms from hanging on for dear life!!!!! We survived but I still have PTSD nightmares from it. LOL ;-) PERSEVERE HONEY

Kathy - Had a bone marrow biopsy too, ouch . . .!!!!! Not expecting to have another for at least 3 more years. I am praying you will not need any marrow transplants - ever! I ran across something I wrote while going through my chemo and thought I'd share it with you. On a piece of paper in my Bible I had written, thank you Lord for letting me live today, help me bless you in it. On the other side of the paper I had written words that I had remembered from a song I'd sung many years earlier. "My life is in your hands and though I may not see clearly, I will lift my voice and sing for your love's an amazing thing. Lord, I know my life is in your hands." Remember, every day is a gift; that is why they call it the present! God is with us moment by moment, that is why His name is "I AM". I'm keeping you and your family in my prayers.

Some Stuff
Jan 23, 2014

Back to the beginning a little. So, because my blood counts are not where they need to be, and my immune system has been all but shut down, I was placed on a Neutropenic diet that consists of no fresh fruit, no fresh vegetables, no flowers, and no pets. No, I don't have pets on the menu, but I can't be visited in my room by them either. I have NEVER wanted a salad so badly in my life, and yet one could kill me. This protects me from bacteria and other infections that could make their way into my shattered immune system that I couldn't fight off if I'd wanted to.

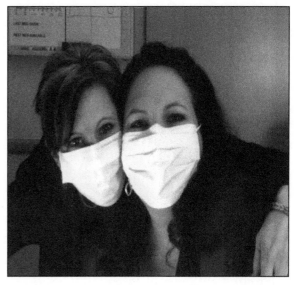

I have also been classified as an "isolated" patient so anyone that enters my room has to have the minimum of a mask, have no signs or symptoms of flu or cold, and sometimes wear a gown. When I leave the room for tests or walks, I have to wear a mask as well. John's even been considerate to shower after wrestling and change his clothes before he comes over. It makes my heart so happy that a middle school kiddo would do that for me. It sucks but is necessary and I'm blessed the people in my life understand these measures and are more than willing to keep me healthy. I do feel bad for them though, especially that first time they burp with the mask on...EVERY single one of them have said they'll never do that again! Funniest thing I've ever seen. Makes me laugh, them not so much.

My nursing team are angels and miracle workers. I don't know where to start with them because there would be too much but might start writing about them individually more as I have time.

And along those lines of time. I thought at the beginning of this that I would have lots of bed time and be reading or doing puzzles or stuff like that. The truth is that reading, and puzzles and games actually hurt my brain. Literally they give me headaches. And for you Candy Crush people out there, I have played one game and not again since January 6th. NO LIE. It's probably for the best... "Candy Crush" is like Crack and I had to go through serious rehab to let it go. I don't recommend this particular rehab to anyone though. Keep playing you Candy CRACK addicts.

Julie - Glad to hear you can have visitors now, seeing people in person is always a nice change! Open your shades today, it's a beautiful sunny day!
Mary - Praying for you, Jenn!!!! Hope you are able to find some foods that still taste good to you even though they aren't fresh. What a bummer!

Emotional roller coaster
Jan 24, 2014

I've been told that between the chemo and the support drugs and the steroids that I may be a bit emotional. That's like saying the sun is a little hot. Holy crap. It's like nothing I've ever experienced before. Tears for no reason. And yes, giggles too. God knew exactly what he was doing when he put the people in my life when he did. I would be a mess if it weren't for the uniqueness of every single person in my life with exactly the "thing" I need at that moment. They bring peace, and prayer, and uplifting notes, and "likes" on Facebook, and Bronco Championship T-shirts, cute hats for my bald head (which isn't yet!), and rubber band bracelets, and boxing gloves, and sort my paperwork, and bring dinner 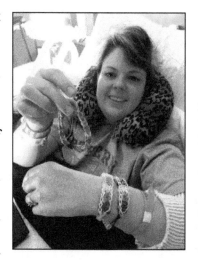 (because I have a stupid craving), and lotion, and movies, and massages, and smiles, and clean laundry, and my special blankie, and a different perspective.....

It's by the grace of God I have you.

Julie - Thanks so much for sharing. I am thinking of you often!
Melissa - You are so special.
Rex - I hope & pray that you've reached the bottom of this chemo treatment curve & the recovery phase will kick into full gear! THANK GOD HONEY...we'll keep on

16

keeping on till u kick this damn leukemia crap in the ass permanently & forever!!!!!
All my love, DAD

Kristin - I tried to bring you a cold Bud light, a Joe look alike stripper, and 50 shades of grey but hospital security drank the bud light, kept Joe the stripper and I got all distracted by the stupid book. Maybe I should stick to dentistry. We love you and miss you.

Karen - Our entire family are saying prayers for you. This, I'm sure, would create different emotions in us all. The Broncos will win and so will you...God is listening! Love you

Update....

Margaret - Jan 26, 2014

Had such a great visit with Jenn on the phone yesterday. She has had a very good two days and is finished with the second round of chemo. We laughed and chatted about the new everyday things...chemo, hospital "stuff", the fabulous food Joe and John are enjoying, etc. OK, so here is vintage Jenn: "I'm not worried about my hair falling out. Now I won't have to shave my legs for a while. That's awesome!" Yes, she said this. Holy cow...talk about seeing the glass half full.

We also talked about the incredible people who have made the difference in how she lives her new "normal." She is profoundly grateful and in awe of the love, kindness and compassion of the people in her life. I guess it's true that what you put out there in the world comes back to you when you need it most. Jenn's positive, upbeat spirit in spite of this illness is both inspiring and deeply humbling. She stood by me steadfastly during some very dark days in my life a while back and I would do anything to take this experience away from her. She adds an entire new meaning to the word "friendship". I am so grateful to all of you who continue to bolster her spirit with posts, actions, and prayers. We stand united next to Jenn until this tempest is over and she is again healthy and well.

Joan - Thank you, Margaret. I think we are united in purple love for you, Jenn.

Rene- Although I don't know you personally, I know you through your parents. I can see you have great faith and a strong will plus a wonderful family. I continue to pray for you and your family.

This Week
Jan 26, 2014

Now three weeks into this, I'm starting to figure out the routine. The initial shock put me in a place of confusion and not understanding vocabulary or treatments and thank Goodness for the daily journal my visitors have helped me put together, I'd feel even more lost. I now understand that the first week of being here were for tests, evaluations, and diagnosis. I then started and just completed an aggressive two-week Chemo regimen that finally ended Saturday and now a week of recovery. I am waiting for my body to begin the most difficult stage of rebuilding what the poison destroyed and create the healthy cells I need to have. I'm on boosters, and transfusions, and anti-everything to make sure my body is protected from even the most miniscule of threat to my destroyed and depleted immune system. Once my levels are healthy and sustainable, I'll be able to go home, probably late this week or early next week. At this point, the "plan", which changes hourly, is to get stable and home for about 3 weeks and then start another 3-week chemo treatment in the hospital again. I'm in this for the long haul.

Today however was the first day of seeing the changes and feeling some of the side-effects of the chemo. I'm tired, not very hungry but eat when I can, and my hair has literally decided overnight to retreat and swoosh. I'll admit I cried in the shower this morning as I watched it go down the drain. But then from seemingly nowhere I was washed over by an amazing sense of strength that helped me realize that these are the signs that the chemo is doing its job on the inside and bringing health back to me. I know it is my faith in moments like these from God that get me through. I feel incredibly blessed to have the ability to mourn, and cry, and openly feel emotions about these things as they come with dignity and sorrow, but can move to a place of peace of knowing I can get past this to what is ahead of me. I believe it was by the Grace of God that I am able to see glasses half full, and potential rather than trouble, and have the perseverance, not doubt, to move on. I thank my God for that blessing, my parents for nurturing it, and everyone else in my life for loving me through this.

I have a feeling this week is going to be full of tests and trials, emotionally and physically, and thank God, I've one big ANGEL TEAM on earth working on my side! Let's get her done!!

Rex - We're with you, Jenn, all the way. Your unbelievable strength of will & character & faith will undoubtedly get you through this. The outpouring of love &

support is a testament to you as a person now & forever!!!!! Love as always, DAD ;-)

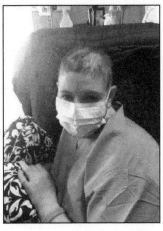

Tammy - Jennifer, your journal entries are truly beautiful and amazing. You are an inspiration to me every day and I look for your thoughts every day. God Bless you and be with you always.

Kathy - I bet you're really cute with your new do ☺ Remember, it isn't your hair that makes you who you are, your beauty comes from within. Jennifer, I hardly know you personally since working pretty much keeps people from really getting to know the persons that work in the same company but are in a different building and we are too busy to get around to know each other. I have kept the little note and life saver that you first gave me when you first began your position here in Weld8. In fact, it was part of my little trinket collection that I keep on my desk until I graduated it into my top desk drawer just last Thursday. Believe it or not, those little gestures of thanks really mean a lot to me. (If you remember, it was a little yellow sticky that had a picture of a bunch of bananas that said "Thanks a bunch! You don't monkey around! then a personal note from you). Wish I could make you feel the way you did to me the day I received your little note. Just want you to know that from the start, I knew you are a beautiful person. And I am glad to be acquainted with you. When I first started the chemo treatments that I had, they told me that the type of medicine may or may not make me lose my hair. I prepared for the worst scenario. I asked my sister that if I went bald I would like for her to paint a Picasso on my head that would point to Jesus all day long. It would remind me and every that worried about me that my life is only because of Jesus and His grace. I am praying for you every day. You come to my mind often and I always lift you to God who is the GREAT PHYSICIAN! He loves you more than anyone can! Keep on keeping on!

Suzanne - Your inner strength and courage is no surprise to me. This is what you taught your students. You are absolutely right, the grace of God is an amazing humbling tool that He gives us. I know you are incredibly beautiful with your new look, because it is always the beauty of the person who shines through. Remember it's the heart that God created first, He knows what He is doing, and you are no exception. You're an inspiration to this family as always. you can do this, and I know your Bronco heart is not going to let this raider reach the next down. Lots of love n hugs. We are here for you just let us know what you need.

Rex - Who needs hair anyway...BALD IS BEAUTIFUL! ;-)

Rose - *Girl you are amazing. I loved hearing your laughter today! I have enough hair for both of us. I cut it off and give it to you any day! <3 U Rosy*

Letting go
January 28, 2014

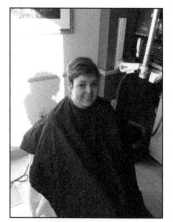

THIS. WAS. HARD. Today was the first time I'd really felt like this was real. And then it was surreal. I had decided long ago that when I started losing my hair I just wanted to shave it off. None of the awkward patchy stuff and why avoid the inevitable. So knowing this was my wish, Stephanie arranged with a hair stylist and the nurses for her to come to my room and take it off. It was such a production with the nurses moving furniture, putting towels down, getting me a chair, having a bag ready to put the diseased hair into. Like a little play of people doing a dance around me. And Ryan, my brother was there. Which I thought was cool because I needed his strength to carry me through this. He doesn't know it, but he is my strength. And then Steph came in with the stylist, both with masks on of course, and I was so excited. Like it was a rite of passage and I was going to be officially knighted into the realm of cancer. When she started the trimmers, I laughed and cried at the same time long with Steph and Ryan. Crying through laughter as she cleared one patch

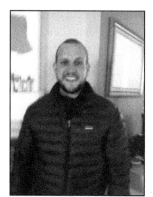
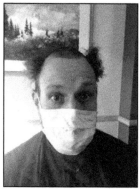

after another. I felt so naked. And so exposed. And very loved. The folks that were there were holding me up and making it possible for me to breathe. When she was done, Steph blurted out "u have a perfect, round head!" and we all laughed again. Then as I got up and they started cleaning things up, Ryan jumped out of his chair and said "my turn!". To say I was shocked would be an understatement, but it meant the world to me. And he did it with such humor and laughter. He allowed the stylist to give him a reverse mohawk. And we laughed and played. He made it light and fun and not the end of the world and I would be ok.

Steph stuck around for a while and had me try on bandanas and hats and did my makeup and took pictures. It was fun to play make-up with her and forget why we were there. It didn't matter. I was letting go of the old and getting ready for the new and clearing a path for the rest of my journey.

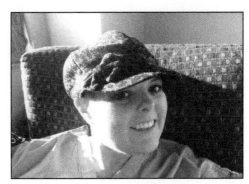

Stephanie
Jan 28, 2014

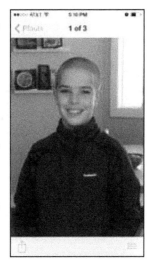

Yesterday was rad and courageous. Jenn had hair falling and surrounding her, as predicted by the aggressive treatment. She made the brave decision to cut it "very short" and stop it from being a nuisance. The hospital set up a nice area with sheets on the floor and a makeshift barber chair. A great stylist named Kim came with her clippers to do the mixed-emotional job of freeing Jenn; from her burdens and her old sickness. Ironically from her own head of hair. The first sweeps were dramatic. As the rest if the hair went, there came a time of trimming and crying and laughing and getting used to a bald head.... the shortest hair she'd had since she was born. She was a champion. Boasted on the Lord the whole time. She was confused at why she wasn't mad, wasn't bitter. It all revealed a fresh head, a renewed spirit, and a gorgeous face that never needed hair anyways. She did it so well that Ryan (baby brother) decided to have his head shaved as well. Way less beauty was revealed. Basically, he should have worn a helmet as a child. Dents and dings, scars. Mis-shapen. It made is all laugh so hard we cried. The male nurse, also bald, was captivated and stayed for the festivities. We tried on new hats, bandanas, scarves. She looks GORGEOUS. No joke. A picture of power, grace, and beauty.

Unpredictably predictable
Jan 29, 2014

I can't believe how fast time gets away from me here. My days are filled with little, inconsistent chunks of time that don't allow for much of anything. Although the routine is somewhat predictable, it is literally an hour by hour experience. What I can count on are "Vital Checks" every 4 hours, interrupting whatever it is I'm doing; sleeping, eating, treatments, everything. I can count on morning meds and breakfast around 8. Then the revolving door begins. I can tell they're coming because I can hear them use the hand sanitizer in the hall and put on masks before knocking on the door. Then doctors, nurses, room service, maintenance, the cafeteria. I am alone very little. I'm waited on hand and foot. Both annoying and cool at the same time. The beeps and buzzers and dings and clicks and bells are driving me crazy. There's this one that sounds like a bird chirping that I want to strangle.

I can't wait to get home.

Rex - Hope you can go home really soon honey! You've paid your dues @ the hospital & you deserve a break from that daily hospital routine...Love ya, DAD ;-)
Jennifer - I loved having you here today. My safe place has always been snuggled in your arms. NOTHING can penetrate the love and protection of a daddy.

Hour by hour
Jan 30, 2014

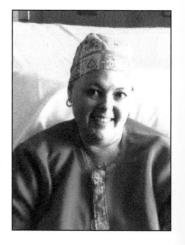

This week has been all about waiting....and patience. Waiting on test results, waiting for reactions or side effects, waiting for my body to shows signs of health, waiting on doctors' reports, waiting. My doctor is hopeful I can be home and on my couch for the Super Bowl, but we are both in no hurry to send me home unstable either. Waiting for blood counts to get to a certain number and stay there. It could be an overnight thing, or take a few more days than hoped. Either way, we are waiting.

And I do mean WE. I can't imagine how difficult it is for my doctor to come in here every day knowing we are hanging on to every word he says (even if I have no idea what he's talking about). EVERYTHING hangs on what he knows, his instinct, his experience, and yes, his inability to predict the future. He can never have a concrete answer because things can change so quickly. He is always using my test results to predict what my body will do, but that's still a best guess and hypothesis. I know he doesn't want to disappoint...I mean really...he did deliver the worst news I've ever had. But since then, he's been right on. I also know how hard he is working for me. He's researching, reading, contacting colleagues, and creating an hour by hour plan just for me...that can change at any time. So we wait and celebrate all the things that could have happened and didn't, the things we hoped would and did, and the things we'll deal with when they come.

WE are waiting. I actually have a hard time even fathoming what "WE" really means. Of course it's Joe and John waiting for me to get home. My family who are here for me daily. And you. My unbelievable WE team. THANK YOU for waiting with me to get me home and through every step along the way.

Angela - *I really hope that you do get to watch the super bowl at home on Sunday!! If that happens I would love to bring you some green chili to celebrate:) Jeff went shooting with Joe on Monday and it sounds like he misses you tremendously. We love you and can't wait to get to hug you!!*
Rex - *This is undoubtedly the most frustrating & difficult part to endure ... the post-chemo phase of your cancer treatment by trying to get your good blood cells to grow back healthy again & to give you enough strength to go home. We're excited too...but trying to be patient @ the same time! Hang in there, honey... Love ya always & forever, DAD*
Melissa - *What a beautiful posting from a beautiful person. You know we are all waiting with you. Love, mom*
Amy - *Jennifer, everything I read from you is such an inspiration. I'm hanging on to your hope and want to pass your words on to others I know struggling with many health challenges. Life is so much in our attitude and your attitude is so positive and encouraging. I am praying you will be home to watch the Super Bowl, as I know what that would mean to you. But that said, If God has another plan, I am wanting His Will. Hang in there. You're a person to be reckoned with. I hope someday to meet you through my precious friend, your sister, Stephanie.*

Kari - You are simply amazing, Jenn!!! Praying that your body is ready for home soon!!! I will also continue prayers for the WE team! :)

Suzanne - Waiting with you. God's will is an incredible journey when we are patient. Praying that this waiting is a blessing and a miracle all wrapped in together. Big hugs for an incredible inspiring positive woman who is winning just because of her strength and courage.

Broncos baby!
Jan 31, 2014

Michelle took me to the rally with her! She took my sign? Might show up on the Today Show this morning. I feel like I'm right there with her!!

I gotta tell ya. This watching the Broncos from a hospital thing is killing me more than the Leukemia. I've been a Broncos fan since my dad dyed my shoes ORANGE in 1978 when they went to the Super Bowl. I got season tickets with Stephanie in 1996 and as a family, we've been tailgating for nearly 20 years. It was tradition. With the normal changes life sends us, we don't often all get together for games anymore, so when we do, it's really special.

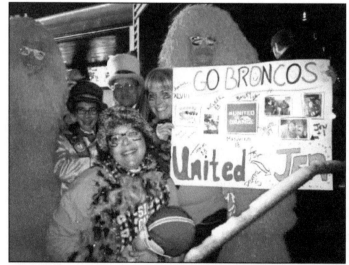

So Stephanie and I have been waiting for this opportunity for 20 years. It's been a bucket list item since before I cared what a bucket list was. It was just assumed that if we managed to get as far as the Big Game again, we would be there come hell or high water. We'd go to all the home games. Go to all the home post-season games. And then find a way to get there. Here's the agony. Steph actually won the ticket lottery and actually got Super Bowl tickets for this year. We are both crushed that such a dream would come true when there's no possible way we can take advantage of it. I am surrounded by Hell and High Water and think I'm feeling the first of many true sacrifices to come.

Paula - *Hi Jenn, just checking in to send you prayers for a fast recovery. You know I live in WA right? I can't be a Bronco fan for you this Sunday. But, if the Broncos win I will think of you and still be happy! Missing you girl!*
Julie - *That's awesome.*
Karly - *I saw this post this morning. Then I happened to see the beginning of the Today show. I just happened to see this poster with your friends. :)*

GOING HOME!
February 1, 2014

I finally got the thumbs up to go home. I'm scared and excited. It's been 30 days since I was in my house. I got up January 6th, got ready for work as though I'd be home later that day, and ended up in the hospital for 4 weeks. I still can't imagine how wrong that was. Life went on at the house without me and I have no idea what I'm going home to. Or how I'll feel. I'm bald. I'm cold all the time. I have no energy. I can't do so many things and I'm really scared of getting sick again. I'm not that naïve to think I'm walking back into normal, but I don't know anything. Period.

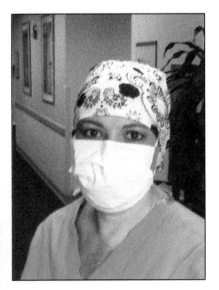

Someone else has been monitoring my every move, every minute. Heart feeds and blood sugars, and hemoglobin and urine output, and sleep and meds. Someone else has been telling me what to do for 30 days. I don't know if I trust myself to take care of myself because I don't know what I'm doing. I feel so clueless.

So I sit here on the edge of the bed waiting for everyone to pick up my meds in the pharmacy, and pack my suitcases (3 of them), and get the release papers, and all of it is going in one ear and out the other. I hope someone is listening.

But I'm going home and I have a care plan and I already know I'll be back to the hospital in less than a week. Which, now that I think about it, being here is normal and comfortable and predictable and I'm scared to go home.

But I'm so happy to be going home and hanging out with my family and Sydney the dog. Home is home and I made it this far.

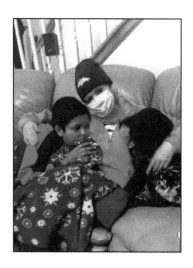 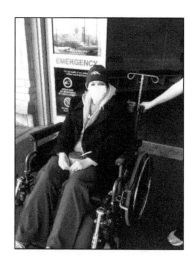

Update!
Margaret – Feb 3, 2014

***Well, despite the Broncos' loss** last night, Jenn is of course 100% behind her team! Disappointed, but there's always next year! She is so happy to be home and has already had a visit from her home health nurse so she can manage her myriad meds, IV's etc. Her blood tests that just came back look great...whew! She goes back in the hospital at the end of the week for round 2 of her chemo treatments and will be there eight to ten days. Things are looking so good though, which is such a relief.*

Rex - God is the QB on Jenn's road to remission team!

Prairie View Middle School Angels
Feb 4, 2014

I can't thank the staff at Prairie View Middle School enough for taking such great care of John and my family during this crazy time. You are truly generous and kind and I appreciate all you've done beyond words.

PVHS Peeps

I'd also like to thank the staff at Prairie View High School for being terrific, enduring friends. Your prayers, thoughts, words of support, love, and continued faith that I can beat this keeps me going.

Ft. Lupton Friends

To all my new friends in Ft. Lupton...

I don't have the words to express how truly blessed I feel to have become a member of the Ft. Lupton family. In the short time we have known each other, you have truly taken me in as one of your own and treated me with love, kindness, and grace. I have NO DOUBT that my positive prognosis has much to do with knowing I will return to a place I love being in and surrounded by people who are genuinely happy to see me. I woke up every day happy to be going to a place where I felt I belonged. And I wake up every day wishing I were there. I miss u all terribly and hope to be back before long. As I go through all this, I am certain it is because of you and your support, and the promise I'll be going back to you, that I will make it through.

Gina - Can't wait to have you back! Sure do miss you!
Jeana - I'm very ready to have you back :). Miss you tons. I'm so glad that you are a part of our family here.

Chapter 2

On the Road Again

Reality hits
Feb 6, 2014

The hardest thing I've ever had to do, next to putting John on the school bus his first day of kindergarten, was wake up this morning. I'm leaving the comfort of my home, husband and son, my couch buddy Sydney, and freedom to purposefully go to a place that is going to break me down to nothing. Again. Today I'm checking back in to the hospital to retake all the invasive tests (bone marrow biopsy, lumbar tap, EKG, etc.) and tomorrow Chemo starts again. And all the things that make the hospital miserable: the food, constant checks by nurses and doctors, having vitals checked all hours of the day and night, a revolving door of people, little peace. Hell part two. I'm having a hard time seeing anything positive today. And finding out yesterday some real truth about the fight I have in front of me is just plain depressing. If I'm lucky enough that my brother or sisters are a bone marrow match, then I can expect 1-2 more rounds of Chemo before a stem cell transplant later in the spring. And then months of recovery, pretty much quarantined until my new immune system kicks in.

At least I can be at home for most of that. (Positive!)

If they aren't a match, it means looking through the bone marrow registry for a donor and a longer wait and more chemo. Best case scenario seems impossible and I don't even want to look past that.

Reality really kicked my butt yesterday and hit me in the face today. And I'm giving myself permission to have a pity party today.

Because: I'm still thankful for my life. I'm thankful for today. I'm thankful for my family and friends who I know will be with me through it all. And I just don't know how to quit. (Positive).

Julie - *Hey girl, stay strong. We are all praying that you find the strength to get through all of this. You are you going to be a stronger person once you get through this. Let me know if you need anything.*

Kari - *Jenn, you are allowed to have a pity party!! I'm thinking of you, praying for you, and sending positive vibes to you!! Hang in there darling!!! I wish I could take this all away!!! I'm going to pray for a bone marrow match and that round 2 goes quickly so you can get back to the comfort of your home!!!*

Rex - *We're with you honey all the way! PITTY POTS ARE CERTAINLY ALLOWED. This is not going to be a picnic but if these treatments can help to get you into a full remission then we'll be with you every step of the way!!!!! Love ya & God bless, DAD*

Lana - *You can do it Jen. Prayers are with you always* 😍

Suzanne - *Girl you are doing great! Facing reality with your strength and positivity is incredible. I don't believe it's a pity party, I'm a true believer it's a natural response to a very unnatural circumstance. All will be ok. Although times are tough, you have an incredible support system full of love. I am thankful for your courageous heart releasing its pain. So that you and your body can use all energy to get well. I am here for you if I can help in any way. Big hugs and lots of love,*

Julie - *Ugh. It's a process with lots of ups and downs. Just know that when you're down there is an up right around the corner. We are here for you. My friends' son just won the battle after 4 Years of fighting cancer. You can do it too! Hugs.*

Amy - *I love that you can vent (be real) and then do what you need to do. So many people are behind you and need to hear your feelings so they can pray specifically for you. I can't imagine being in your shoes. Thank you for your honesty. I'm praying.*

Mary - *Jenn, my heart goes out to you. You are in the worst of it right now. Try to picture yourself one year from now. You will be healthy, back at home for good, and a stronger woman who beat cancer. It is your nature to be a positive and happy person and I believe in you. Hang in there - this is a battle worth fighting.*

Michelle - *Thinking of you Jen and sending prayers your way. Please know that I'm watching out for John each day at school trying to be support for him.*

Settling in
Feb 7, 2014

So now that I'm here, unpacked, and settling in, I'm doing ok. At least much better than yesterday. I'm getting used to my "new normal". The good thing is that I'm returning MUCH stronger than I came in the first time and have the motivation and strength to really fight and beat this. I also know the routine and things aren't a mystery this time; I know what to expect and don't feel lost. It was also great to be able to pack what I wanted to bring this time. It's amazing how that little bit of control can make such a huge difference.

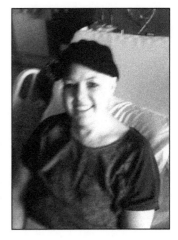

Knowing this time what comforts from home to bring made a huge difference right from the beginning. I brought my lamp again. I can't tell you how important that was. Everyone noticed it when they walked in because it was such a relaxing light versus the fluorescent nuisance options that were just obnoxious. I also brought pictures from home, a lot of comfortable sleeping clothes and underwear, my own blanket and pillow and my journal. That was critical for me, my memory, and the doc's and nurses. Lotion, lip gloss, and air freshener too. It made my room much less sterile and a lot more like home.

I flew through my first day of treatment today without reactions or side effects and am ready for tomorrow. My blood counts came in better than expected and doc is really pleased with the results. This stay looks to be 8-10 days with the possibility of going home as early as next Friday or Monday after another Lumbar Tap. It's so day by day. I'm learning a lot of patience!

It looks like a stem cell/bone marrow transplant is a definite and will keep me busy with recovery well into the summer. The hope is that one of my sisters or brother will be a match, but not a guarantee. It would take place later this spring, with a long stretch of isolation while my new immune system takes over. And that's IF a family member is a match. If not, I go into the registry and hope for a match from a non-related donor. Because of my rather simple genetic makeup (white female with an uncomplicated generic background) a match looks promising. Again, patience is a requirement.

Still feeling blessed by the outpouring of love and support for me and my family. I am certain the prayers and positive thoughts are a tremendous part of my success so far. Keep 'em coming!

Rex - _Your attitude inspires me to be a better person & shows me how much of a warrior you really are! There's no doubt in my mind that your courage & grit will help get you through this battle w/ leukemia! Love you now & forever, DAD_
Mary - _Feeling stronger than when you started, and your blood counts are better than expected...YAY! I hope this week slips by quickly._

Next...
Feb 13, 2014

So... Part 2 of cycle 1 is over and it really kicked my butt. Not the actual Chemo - I can handle the headaches and soreness - but the treatment itself is brutal. I had 2 nights of constant checks for blood glucose levels (finger pricks), Ph levels (urine tests), chemo blood levels, premeds to prepare for the chemo, the chemo itself which also required a "neuro check" which meant numbers and

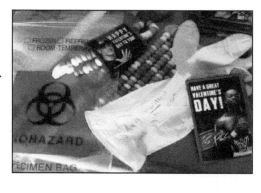

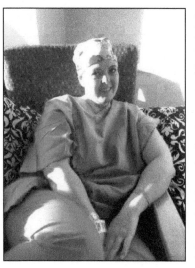

getting out of bed, beeping machines, poking, prodding, and NO SLEEP. And of course none of this could be timed better so I could get more than 30 minutes of sleep. REALLY? I was miserable. But after a good nights' sleep and my tests looking good, it seems I'll be going home tomorrow afternoon - just in time for Valentines' Day! My good friend noted that holidays seem to be the goal; the Super Bowl, Valentine's Day, and if my calculations are correct, after my next treatment I could be home for St. Patrick's! HAHAHAHA! This stay at home will be about 2 weeks and will be accompanied by 2-3 in-patient tests a week and possible transfusions. But I'll

32

be HOME! For 2 weeks! I can't tell you how excited I am for that. I will be able to sleep and the constant monitoring will go away.

I also experienced new emotions this week that are hard to deal with. I've only been out of the hospital 10 days this ENTIRE YEAR. Since January 6th there are so many things I took for granted that I haven't been able to do...drive a car, go to the store, be with people, work, hug people without a mask on, go to the bank (get gas, the cleaners, drive throughs, etc.). I haven't been able to watch John wrestle or tuck him in at night. And I haven't nudged Joe in the middle of the night telling him to roll over because he's snoring. All these things will return in time, but it's been hard to accept.

It's also been hard to watch life go on for everyone else. Every time I'm included on an email from work, I'm not only happy to feel included, but also sad that things are rolling along without me. On the one hand I can take credit for getting things to a place where they are self-sufficient, people are empowered to step up, and the wheels aren't falling off. On the other, will they need me? It's a bit of a pity party attitude that I'm syoure I'll shake, but it is my reality for now.

Other news: Steph, Becky, and Ryan all completed their tests to see if they are a match for my stem cell transplant. The results should be take 3-4 weeks (I am frustrated it might take that long), and then we can start the process for a transplant if they are a match. If they aren't, then we go to the registry and possibly have donor drives to see if any of you are a match. You never know...one of you may be my perfect match (internally) and we never knew it! But cross your fingers it's one of my sibs so I can get the recovery of 100 days of progressively less isolation - at home - over. It'll be hard, and I still have to complete the second round of Chemo (both parts), but that's the goal. Cross your fingers and keep praying.

Rex - We're all thrilled you will have a couple of weeks @ home trying to enjoy your "new normal". Of course, we'll be available for out-patient trips back & forth to the Hospital & to help w/ tasks in & around the house. Much love honey, DAD
Me - Ang, watching you stand at the door and watching you through the stairs (jail bars) not being able to hug you killed me too. I cried after you left. Hopefully after this week at home I can have visitors! I'll be home until the first week of March. We love the breakfast burritos and those are good for breakfasts for the boys. And the muffins! MmmmmMmmmm. Side dishes like mac and cheese, baked potatoes, salads, and fruit is awesome. LOVE YOU!!

Rose - Leaders empower others to step up just as you have those you work with. They need you...they know that. Your focus is you and your health! After reading Ang's message I am selfishly glad I can't get rid of this cold. I couldn't stand in the door and not hug you. VIRTUAL hug girl! <3 & prayers

Tammy - Continued prayers for you. I am already on the marrow registry. I've been on it for 10 years and have never been called. Maybe I will be your match. Praying like crazy that one of your siblings are a perfect match for you.

Kim - So glad you will be home for Valentine's Day. Prayers are continuing.

Angela - I cried too :-). It's so hard to think that we can't just grab a beer and have a bitch session like the old days!! Soon we will. I will definitely make some food and can't wait to be able to deliver it directly to you. I think a pan of cheesy potatoes is in order. We love you so much and you inspire us every day.

Todd - Best wishes to you girl! We're praying for you often and keeping the good vibes coming your way.

Suzanne - Jennifer, praying for many miracles and many matches. I am available if needed for a match testing. You keep hanging in there. This is not an easy time of life, but there will come a time when you look back and say, "I made it!" There are many celebrations along the way. You can do this. I am proud of you for speaking truthfully about every step along the way. Releasing the feelings both good and bad are healthy for you. I pray every day for great news to come your way. Hugs my friend.

Going home
Stephanie Downing Feb 14, 2014

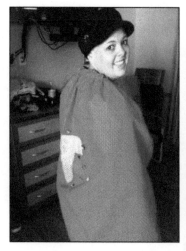

Last day here for a while! Yay! They are loading her up with meds so she can have an extended stay at home. It may be up to two weeks before she is re-admitted! She spent the day making Valentine bags to thank her nurses and care team. They had wrestler valentine notes that said, "Thanks for being in the fight with me," and candy necklaces, and rubber gloves that said, "You have HANDled me with care." Hehe. She packaged them in bio-hazard bags. Hilarious. This afternoon she put on her cape and went to deliver some love. Only Jennifer, the patient, is able to bring such joy and sunshine to a floor that needs so much hope. Amazing! Check out the pictures!

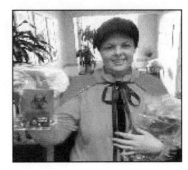

Surprised em' again!!
Feb 17, 2014

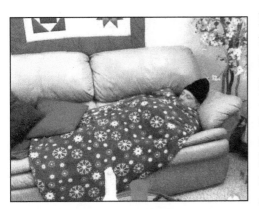

I went into the chemo and transfusion clinic today to see how I did over the weekend (blood counts). Apparently, I didn't just do good, I knocked it out of the park. Although I'm now officially neutropenic again (immune system broken and can't handle anything), my other blood counts were again higher than they expected and .... No blood transfusion for me!!! Woohoo!! My blood is doing its thing and I didn't need the "boost" they expected I would. The nurse even said, *"Aw, all grown up and making blood all by yourself!"* Joe almost fell out of his chair he was laughing so hard. I cried. It's been a good day.

Now I need to focus on staying away from anything my immune system can't handle: infection, virus, bacteria, pneumonia, and anything that could attack my system or organs. Hopefully this should last less than a week as my body starts creating the white blood cells I need. CAUTION is the name of the game now.

And I can't say it enough; I couldn't do this without the love and support of my family, friends, and each and every person praying and sending me positive vibes. I'm not doing this alone. Just when I start feeling down or start allowing myself to think negatively, one of you comes through with something that cheers me right up or puts me in a better place. I can't do it without you.

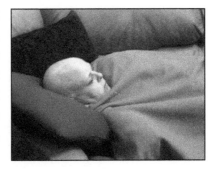

Rex - HOORAY...good report! Now we need to keep you away from infections of any kind. See ya soon ;-) Love ya, DAD
Rene - Congratulations, Jennifer! Prayer is a wonderful thing.
Mary - Wow Jennifer - Life is good! Your poor body has been so much, yet it is coming through for you. Is there a way people can donate blood so that you get credit for it, so to speak?

Being Back
Mar 5, 2014

Forgive me for not updating while I was at home. There really wasn't much to update. It was a rather uneventful 2 weeks of snuggling with my boys, watching movies, doing some things around the house, and glorious 8-10 hours of nightly (QUIET and UNBOTHERED) sleep. I had appointments every other day to check my counts, and I loved every minute of getting out and around. And on one of the last days, my sister Stephanie took me out to a belly-busting lunch in which we got to watch some guys at the club house drink and have conversations that should never be repeated, and yet the bar tender told us they were just getting started. We took away many one-liners that still set us off into hysterics. Bacon, meat coolers, 6am beers, and missing teeth. Yep...I'm chuckling now.

I checked back in yesterday for Cycle 2, Part 1, (I didn't cry this time) and now know why people hate going to the hospital, or the doctor for that matter. I forgot how loud it is here. The nurses' phones constantly ringing and with different ring tones, the machines beeping all with different tones and urgencies, the call buttons, the beeps of nurses getting into locked/restricted doors, the people walking up and down the hall, the music when a baby is born (always brings a smile), and the music to remember to turn over (Turn, turn, turn - also brings a smile). And the ridiculous restrictions - they REALLY DO make a person feel sick in here. And some doctors just don't listen. To me, to nurses, to anyone. Now, Dr. Hyde - my oncologist - is amazing and is truly a partner in my care. The other folks labeled my general practitioners are a joke. The guy who came in yesterday ordered treatments I don't need and clearly didn't look at my previous charts. He's as bad or worse than the dr. I went to in January whose diagnosis was anxiety and sent me home with a prescription for anxiety meds...until she saw my bloods test results and whisked me off to the ER. REALLY? This new and temporary Dr. of the day and I will have a little chat next time I see him. For those of you who know me well, I know you're already feeling a little sorry for him. Don't. I can be gentle when I want to be. :-)

It was strange walking through these very familiar 5th floor halls and being not only greeted by the nurses with smiles but being called out by name as though seeing an old friend. Many of them came to my room to say hi and see how my family and I were doing. It was like we all forgot the reason I was here was to save my life, but it didn't matter. I have a superb team of nurses and CNA's that have made my treatments as tolerable as possible and managed to make this my second home as best they can. They know Joe and John and my mom and dad and siblings and ask how they are all doing. And they listen to the answers. It may be possible I'll miss these people once this is all said and done.

And as I look for positives, they are easy to find. Things are going great so far; better than expected is what I hear. I'm starting this cycle stronger and healthier than I have been for months. Dr. Hyde calls me a young whipper-snapper whose body is just waiting to take over and get better. My numbers are high, I'm not seeing the side effects I could be, and this will be another short 10-12 day visit with the probability of going home next Friday. AND... with the assistance of Netflix, I'm catching up on all the shows I should have been watching all along: Orange is the New Black, Breaking Bad, House of Cards, 24, and the list goes on. I have a gorgeous view from my window. The extent of the people sending positive thoughts and prayers are far beyond my ability to comprehend and I believe the reason I am doing so well. Again, I am blessed.

Joan - *And YOU are a blessing to us. Showing strength and courage and humor and kindness and that positive spirit. God continues to be with you. Hugs to you.*
Jill - *Get it, rock star! Stay strong. Stay positive! If you haven't watched Orange is the New Black, catch it on Netflix. Love ya, sister!*
Kathy - *Keep that beautiful smile going! It is kind of like a "SON" beam. It helps everyone, even the doctors see Jesus in you! It helps you be the kind of 'rock star' that has their feet firmly planted on "The Rock"! I'm still praying for you (I have you as a prominent yellow sticky by my computer at the office).*
Kari - *You are amazing, Jenn! Love and prayers always!!!*
Rex - *Love ya Jenn - Keep on truckin' honey...I'm really confident that you're going to beat this damn insidious disease! DAD*

Mary - A friend who is in more than 15 years of remission after stage 4 breast cancer goes to an annual potluck at her hospital in South Denver. The get together in January to kick off a new year of remission and friendships. The bonds you form with your healthcare professionals and sometimes other patients can last a lifetime. A l-o-n-g- lifetime! You are in a battle, but you are not fighting it alone Jenn! I hope these next few days pass quickly for you.

Jeana - Loved reading your update. I wish I could somehow overhear the same bar conversation, they sound HILARIOUS, lol!!!!! You ARE a young Whipper Snapper, by the way... it shows in every word of your posting. Keep it up. We are rooting for you in Fort Lupton!!!!

Shirley - Hi Jennifer, Glad to hear you are fighting through this. Know that Warren and I are praying for you to have a full recovery and see you back in school. If you need anything, please let me know. Thanks and God bless you!

Rex - We're IN IT 2 WIN IT ... w/ you all the way honey! Love you now & forever, DAD

Voodoo Donuts
March 6, 2014

So Voodoo Donuts just opened in Denver and I've never had one, but everyone says they're amazing. For some stupid reason I couldn't get them out of my mind, and that's remarkable considering everything tastes like crap. So a few days ago I called my brother to see if he could get me some. He said he was on a 30 cleanse and would love to when he's done. But yesterday I got the funniest voice message EVER from him. I'm going to

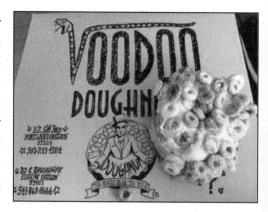

transcribe it, but I'm sure it won't be the same without the pure torture in his voice. He was really suffering, but I still laugh hysterically when I listen to it.

(March 5, 2014 – Ryan voicemail)
Alright. It's eight o'clock on Wednesday... and I'm on day 10 of my cleanse... and I'm feeling great, I have tons of energy, I'm eating well, I'm running, I'm

exercising. However. Since you brought up Voodoo Donuts I cannot stop thinking about Voodoo Donuts and dreaming about donuts and 6-pound donuts that I want to eat. Donuts. Fried, dough. Dough in my mouth…Donuts. I'm so mad. I'm hangry. That's…that's what I… I mean…Hangry is the best word for what I am right now. I want a cream filled piece of fried dough…topped with…chocolate and, sprinkles…. maybe then covered in bacon. I don't know. I might throw some bacon on there because why wouldn't you throw bacon on fried dough stuffed with CREAM (very emphatic)??? Soooo...thanks for that. Hope you're doing well. Love you. Bye.

Let's Talk Showers
March 10, 2014

For years I have stepped into the warmth of a shower and thanked God, literally, for the hot water, my home, and all the blessings that that shower represented. But taking a shower at the hospital is truly a tedious necessity that I dreaded. First, with the help of a nurse, I had to wrap my PICC line so no water could get into the port and create an infection. Then I wheeled in my medicine pole and undressed the best I could. Next we had to lie down towels on the floor so I wouldn't slip and a towel on the bench. The bench, by the way, was the BEST thing ever! I loved to sit on that bench and let the warm water literally wash away the cancer, and my hair, and the nasty Bio-something-or-another soap I had to use to prevent infection, I think. It was then that I again give thanks for the hot water and my life and even the ridiculous process of taking a shower. Somewhere, someone was praying to God they would get one…ever.

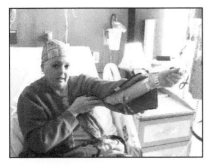

Showers were also hard because the only mirror in the place was in the bathroom, and every time I looked into that mirror, I didn't recognize the person looking back at me. Who is that bloated, bald, broken person? Surreal can't come close to explaining how weird the whole experience was. But showers were the only time I really looked in the mirror and had to admit it was me. I cried a lot in the shower. Good and bad tears. Happy and sad. Praying and exhausted. Hopeful and scared. But always renewing and cleansing.

The process was much friendlier at home because I didn't have to roll my pole in, and I found a cool waterproof "sleeve" I could put over my PICC. And I could again count my blessings.

But I do miss that bench!!

BIG, SUPER FUN EVENT TO BENEFIT THE VENEGAS FAMILY!

Margaret - Mar 16, 2014

Hey, all! *Please mark your calendar...great people, music (Something Underground...incredible band you will not want to miss), food, venue AND a GREAT cause! If you have something to donate to the raffle, please contact Angela who will gladly take your contribution. If you cannot attend, please donate whatever you can! Let's show Jenn and her family tons of love!*

Love, Live, Laugh- Benefit Jenn

Jenn was diagnosed with Acute Lymphocytic Leukemia in January and we are working to raise money to help out the Venegas family. Any donation is appreciated!! We are also holding a benefit March 29th

YOUCARING.COM

Chapter 3

Traveling Through

Hills and Valleys

Transitions
Mar 19, 2014

So, I made it in and out of the hospital for the third time and again didn't have anything really to share. What I realized is that I am in transition between 2 different "new normals": The one at the hospital, and the one at home. They are both so different and yet so alike, but both have started to become routine.

At the hospital it's the routine of starting around 8am (give or take an hour or so) with vitals, meds, and the schedule for the day (tests, treatments, rest, etc.). Then visits from the doctors to go over the test results and see how I'm feeling. There was one day of this when I had 3 people standing around my bed, who had all asked the exact same question, when my regular doc came in and started the inquiry all over. The people already in the room laughed as I told the doc to get an update from one of the other 3 people who had just put me on the witness stand. We joked about putting a dry erase board on my door with those questions on it so people can read it before coming in. Over the top, maybe, but I would have loved it. I never want to hear the following questions ever again:

* *How did you sleep*
* *How do you feel*
* *Have you eaten today*
* *Have you pooped today*
* *Can I get you anything*
* *Do you have nausea, pain, mouth sores, headaches, bruising, rashes, blurry vision, numbness in fingertips or toes, fever, and on and on...*

Throughout the day the vitals continue every 4 hours (but within a 2-hour time frame so anytime really), the meds and treatments, and meals. Now it might sound like this isn't a whole lot, but I also knew I didn't have chunks of time longer than 30 minutes without the anticipation of being interrupted or disturbed, so starting a phone conversation or book or movie or any other task to occupy my time was hard to do. And there was SO MUCH hurry up and wait I could barely stand it... remember, it was totally unpredictable when things were going to happen so I couldn't fill the time with activities either. I gazed out the immense west facing window watching beautiful sun rises and sets, watching the weather come down the slopes and engulf the Boulder Flatirons, and watch the windmills on the hills. I prayed and meditated, a lot, and tried to find peace. Sometimes I could even convince myself that my little room with bed and lamp, and bathroom, and tv, and comfy chairs was actually a hotel room and I was taking a little vacation. I also had many moments of wishing I could be anywhere but there, and sometimes the reality of what I was really there for, hit hard. I HAVE CANCER and I'm feeling the side-effects and having reactions to all the poisons and chemicals my body was being filled with and this is "Normal".

My second normal has been coming home and trying to rejoin the little tribe of men that has done such a remarkable job of taking care of themselves and each other while I was gone. Their routines also changed as mom wasn't there to have dinner ready (or even think to that step in the first place), do the shopping, the laundry, and all the other little tasks they had perhaps never realized mom just took care of. But they did it. John is such a mature young man now and so capable of taking care of himself I really shouldn't have worried about him at all. And Joe is a grown ass man that can also take care of himself. It looked different and dinner was often "pop up and get your own", but they made it work.

Now mom comes back and struggles with how to re-enter her life with her family. And to resume the second-natured things she once did so willingly and lovingly.

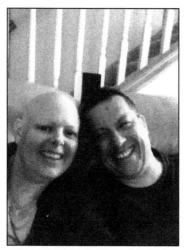

But now mom can't do those things either: cooking and cleaning and laundry and picking up and shopping and making appointments for John or getting him rides. And they still have to get done. And when can she speak up and when should she let things go? And resisting the urge to do them anyway but knowing it's not part of the "recovery and get stronger" plan. I sometimes admit I feel like a stranger here and try to fit in as much as possible. They watch their tv shows, have their inside jokes, wrestle and are, in general, perfectly capable of doing it on their own.

My routine of Normal now has to concentrate on making sure I take my meds (and remember to do so 3-4 times a day), drink enough water, eat, rest, schedule appointments and find rides to get lab work done 3 times a week. I get so overwhelmed and my brain literally hurts, but it has to get done too.

And trying to help Joe and John into my new world is a difficult transition too. This is after all my fight and there's no possible way they can relate to what I'm going through. But they also have to live with the outcome and in every way the things that affect me. I struggle with how much do they need to know: the details of the diagnosis, and the side effects I'm having, and how involved with the appointments should they be. And I don't want to scare them, or push too much on them, or leave them out of anything. It's like I told John at the very beginning of all this: "I've never been through this before and there's no instruction manual, and I don't know what to expect or how to react to it, and I'm going to do the best I can." We're all doing the best we can and surviving this together.

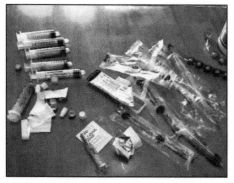

And this is part of my daily routine. Joe has to "flush" my PICC line and it takes all this to do so. Alcohol swabs, syringes, caps for the PICC line. The blood thinner followed by several syringes of saline to keep the line open. We joke about it now like it's a strange and funny dating ritual or foreplay. It's become a nice time to connect and talk and giggle. It's interesting how that's our new normal.

Although this journal may seem less positive as others, that's not the case at all. I'm being reflective and letting things settle in as they come. And have NO DOUBT I am going to kick this thing and do so with the support and love of my family, creating yet another normal.

Gail - What A Touching Journal. I Think You Should Write A Book For Others. You Are An Amazing Lady And I Love You. Gail
Mary - Such a mixed blessing, Jennifer. Your tribe of men are adapting to your being away. Bless you for allowing us a glimpse into your life and I now have a better understanding of why they call it a "battle" against cancer. I can't wait to see you at the LLL celebration and fundraiser on the 29th. Meanwhile, maybe we can bring you a small white board to write your list of questions on, with a place to check yes or no!
Rex - We have absolutely NO DOUBT that you will have a full & complete recovery from this insidious disease. Love you now & forever, DAD
Tasha - Jennifer, the Chicago-faction of the family is sending our love and support. Tiffany (two my kids), Jac and Tim, (niece) Hope, (ma and hubby) Karen and Paul and (my brother) Kevin - we love you!
Robert - Dear Jennifer, I'm sorry I'm so late in writing you, but have just now figured out how to write you a message. Barbara and I are two of the gang that your mom and your siblings invited to your Dad's surprise 50th birthday party in May 1994. We have been following your story and admire your strength, knowing that his is a very wearing time. You are always in our thoughts and prayers. Love, LeRoy and Barb

She's a match!
Mar 27, 2014

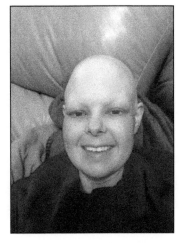

The magic words I've been waiting to hear for months now have finally been spoken and are a reality!! My sister Becky is a bone marrow match and we go for a transplant during Holy Week (April 13)! This process has been long and patience has been necessary, but we're a go. Becky had to undergo an extensive regimen of tests and examinations for us to get to this point, but she's in perfect health and ready to fork over a ridiculously large amount of her marrow (about 2-3 small wine bottles - I didn't know that was possible...) for me to adopt as my own. I've spent the last week and will spend the next two weeks having tests of my own, many duplicated from the very beginning (CAT, ECHO, bone marrow biopsy, lumbar tap, x-rays, EKG, etc.). AND THANK YOU TO MY ANGEL TEAM OF TAXI DRIVERS WHO HAVE MADE IT POSSIBLE TO MAKE THE APPOINTMENTS - Mom, Dad, Michelle, and Annie.

Al Michaels once said, *"Do you believe in miracles?"* as the US Men's Olympic Hockey team beat the Russians and then went on to win the Gold Medal in the Olympics. Yes, I believe in miracles and I believe they happen all the time, randomly and planned, big and small, with and without notice. Before January, I saw many occurrences I would call miracles simply because I couldn't explain how they happened. I've seen students pull off graduation in a mad, 1-2-day rush. I've come within inches of disaster more times than I want to admit - mostly because I stupidly made bad choices that put me in those positions in the first place. And if you're a Broncos fan, you'll know the Tebow season in general was a miracle. :-) Whether you want to call them miracles or blessings, I've been the benefactor of many more than my share in this life, let alone in the past 3 months. And I now believe there's no such thing as big or small miracles. They're all ginormous to the people they happen to because it's all about each person's perspective and reality.

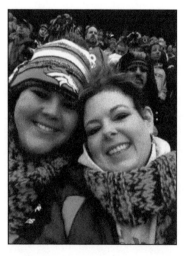

Becky has been a miracle since she was born. And I believe this path for both of us was planned way before that. We knew the minute they said "bone marrow transplant" and "siblings" that she would be a match. I don't know how we knew...we just did. It was like putting that one, tricky puzzle piece, in the only place that made the whole puzzle come into focus. It just fit. And she's saving my life. She's been on board since the very beginning and is willing to undergo a painful procedure to harvest the cells. She's now my own personal miracle and I'll never be able to repay her for saving my life.

And it's not a coincidence or irony to me that the actual process is taking place during Holy Week. On Holy Thursday, while Chemo and Radiation is killing my bone marrow and stem cells (those little bastards that would now identify the cancer

46

cells as friends and let them back in to the party if they were to knock on the door), my sister will be sacrificing her own to replace mine. As her cells are transfused into me, I'll be going through the process of literally rebuilding, renewing, and regenerating a whole new me. Becky's strong and healthy bone marrow will overpower my weak stuff and start to produce healthy stem cells, which in turn create the healthy blood, and so on. And these new cells will recognize the "raider" as an enemy and destroy it. I will be experiencing the miracle of a true rebirth during Easter weekend, and praising every blessing, celebration, and miracle that made it possible.

Psalms 126:3 - *And so we celebrated because the Lord had indeed worked miracles for us.*

Tammy - That's awesome news! Miracles do happen. Every. Day. I'm so happy to hear this news!
Todd - That is an awesome irony! Fantastic! Best wishes girl!
Mary - Happy dance in progress!
Janet - Jen, this is wonderful news!! Having known you and Becky since birth, I'm thinking back to so many times that you have supported and helped each other. This is the ultimate support, and I know that Becky gives it with an open heart. I can't tell you how happy this makes me. Lots of love, Janet

Angels
Mar 28, 2014

Lately I've been thinking a lot about all the things that had to fit perfectly into place for me to be in the positive position I'm in. And all the people that have sacrificed, prayed, and acted in a supportive way.

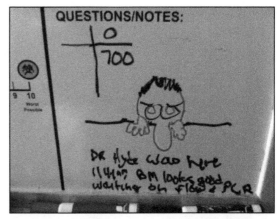

The nurses and doctors at Exempla Good Samaritan Hospital - who have NO idea what they mean to me. They saved my life and although they were annoying at times, I know I COULD NOT have made it through three, 2+ week long treatments without their support. The job is one thing, the heart they brought is quite another. It was a blessing I ended up at that special place.

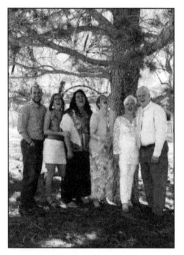

Dr. Hyde - Who went the extra mile EVERY SINGLE day to research, study, and examine every piece of literature and my data and the medications and the treatments and the side-effects before making any decision. And his wonderful demeanor and sense of humor. And for his tireless devotion to the oncology field and his passion for helping people. And for getting up at 4 in the morning to check labs and going to bed at midnight after making rounds. "I only need 4 hours of sleep", he would say. And for saving my life. It was a blessing he was at the hospital that Monday night I checked in.

My Family (Mom, Dad, Stephanie, Becky and Ryan) - who, as we Slaughters do, had a companion/visiting schedule in place before the end of the 2nd day. We come together and sacrifice like no other family I know. Each of my family members had their role and place by my side and were my rocks. Mom and dad who travel the hour and a half drive from Colorado Springs to be here at least once a week. And my siblings who have been everything to me - from shaving their head, to filling out my HR and FMLA forms, to setting up my room with all the things visitors would need (snacks, chargers, blankets and pillows) and doing the things Joe just couldn't get to (meals, folding laundry, shopping). It is a beyond a blessing that I have them.

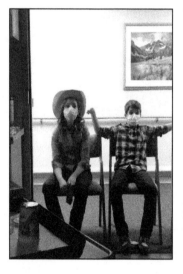

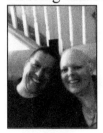

And Joe - who in an instant became mom and dad, and chauffeur, and spectator, and cook, and cleaner, and essentially a single parent. Who is selfless in taking time off for John's activities and appointments or my needs and appointments. Who is my hero. He is a blessing.

And John - who is such an amazing young man. Who also picked up the responsibilities of taking care of himself (laundry, and rides to and from activities, and meals, and the pets) without complaint or question. I honestly don't have the words to express how much I love him and proud of him I am. He is my life and a blessing.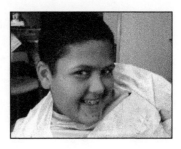

And our colleagues - past and present. Whose support, notes, gifts, meals, prayers, cartoons, and love have fed me and my family throughout this time. I am convinced that had this happened a year ago, I would NOT have the amazing recovery I am having now. It would have been much more difficult to find a reason to fight. Now there is no question in my mind what I need to do to beat this. Not enough can be said about the Colorado State Patrol - who always take care of family, and the Ft. Lupton and Brighton School Districts. You are my blessings.

And the colleagues and friends of my brother and sisters (Stephanie, Becky, and Ryan) - who don't know me from Eve but have adopted me as family because of the love and respect they have for them. It's such a tribute to Steph, Becky and Ryan that their "people", most of them strangers to me, have reached out in support of all of us. Here's a shout out for the folks at American Family, Atlas Management, and Lafayette Elementary. Blessings to me on a whole different level.

And the friends that have stayed the course with me through all this. Who have lived up to their promise to be supportive. Who text daily, post or follow the Facebook and Caring Bridge pages, who have made meals, sent gift cards, provided rides to my appointments, answer the phone no matter the time of day or night, calm my fears, help me focus on the goal, lift my spirits, and who pray (in whatever manner it means to them). For not leaving my side when being a friend was just too difficult now that I have a crisis going on. You have sustained me and are my blessings.

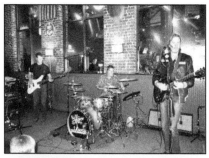

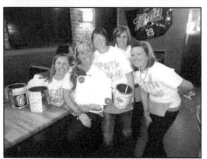

AND TO THE AMAZING ANGEL TEAM - that concocted, schemed, organized, planned, and will pull off the best party ever...in my honor. Angela and Jeff, Michelle, Casey, Kari, and Keeley have walked the streets, made phone calls, created flyers and t-shirts and koozie's, collected donations, brought in a band (Something Underground - who volunteered their evening), and promoted tomorrow's benefit like professionals. They have spent their personal time wrapping t-shirts with ribbon, working out details with the Copper Rail, sorting donations into gift baskets for the auction, and thinking through every last detail - just to help out a friend. I honestly have no idea to what ends they have traveled to make this possible, but I KNOW it is the most authentically graceful, kind, loving, and generous act I have ever been witness to, let alone on my behalf. I am blessed that in my lifetime I am able to witness the goodness of people and the extent they will go to for a friend. There are NO WORDS strong enough to express how thankful I am for these people. I am eternally grateful for these blessings in my life.

It feels awkward saying this, but PLEASE attend the benefit tomorrow. Not for me, but to honor the people who have made it possible. Your presence alone will let them know their efforts are appreciated and worthwhile. And they deserve every bit of love and support you can give.

Joan - *This beautiful post is so you... always thinking and appreciating others. Looking forward to tomorrow night! God's blessings to you.*
Angela - *We love you Jenn and each of knows you would have done the same for us.*
Casey - *We love you so much and know you would do nothing short of the same to help out anyone if they needed it!*
The Benefit party - *What amazing hands are at work. I honestly can't believe the capable efforts of your friends, Jenn. You are surrounded by people who are kind, loving and selfless in giving of their time and talents. I can't wait for us to hear the beautiful stories that emerge at tonight's benefit! Amazing.*
Mary - *Incredibly kind and thoughtful post, Jenn - so YOU! We are looking forward to this evening and to seeing you.*

Kathryn - That was beautiful, Jenn. I love you and miss you so much. You are strong and can beat this cancer!

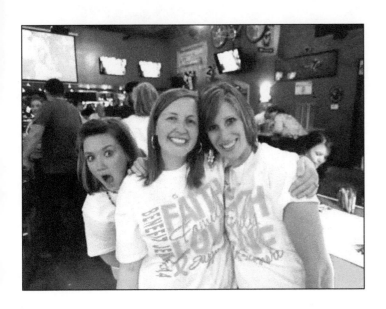

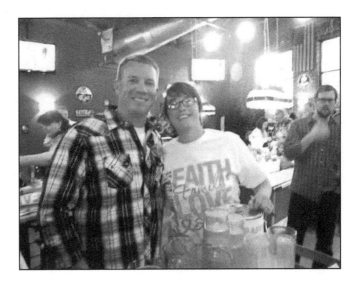

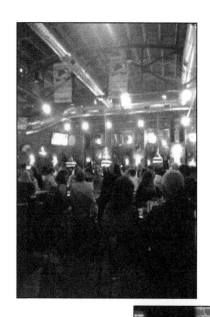

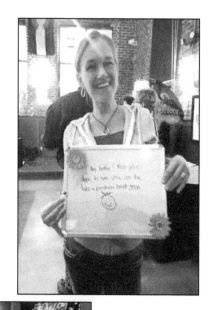

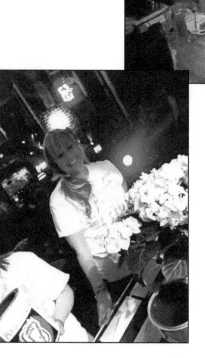

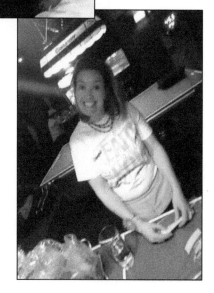

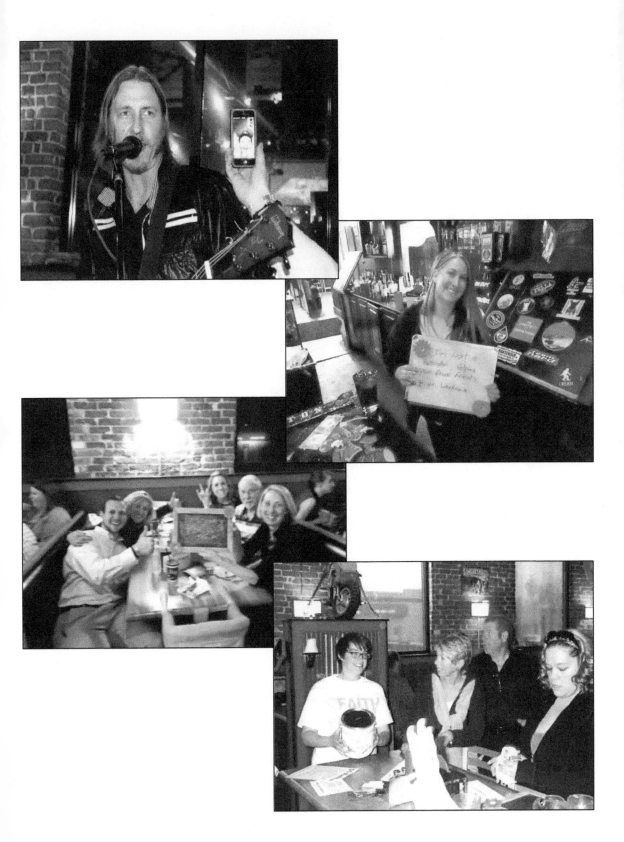

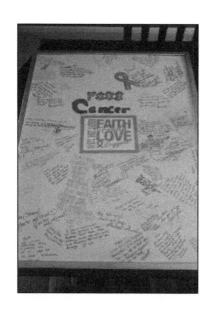

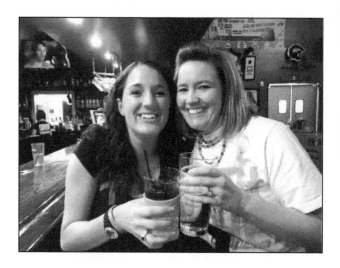

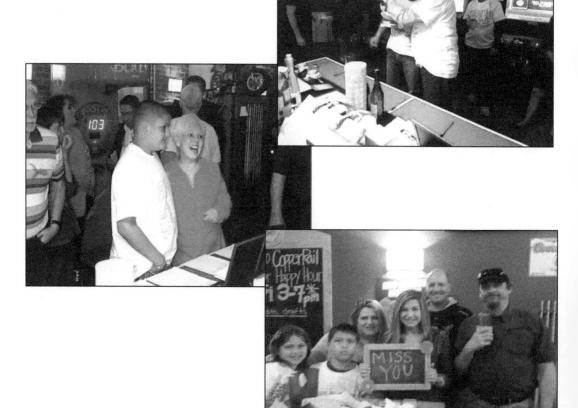

March 31, 2014

<u>Humbly, I want to thank</u> everyone who planned, attended, donated, volunteered, or contributed in any way to this spectacular event. Your generosity is incredible.

Although I couldn't attend in person, my family and friends were there in full force and face-timed me many times making me feel like an active participant. You all were beautiful to see and I'm honored. Your friendship, faith, and support are enduring and inspire me to stay strong and fight this battle.

And thank you for celebrating and loving on my sister Becky as my donor. Her journey will be difficult and painful, and yet she is more than happy to endure this for me. She is my savior and hero and I cannot say enough about her courage and love.

On to the next phase...Transplant and hopefully Long-Term Remission! More to come.

Thank you
Apr 6, 2014

On behalf of Joe and John, we'd like to sincerely thank all the wonderful people who made such generous donations. We are overwhelmed by and eternally grateful, more than we could ever show, for your thoughtfulness and support during this time of uncertainty and apprehension. Your caring gift will help us with the medical bills and other daily expenses we will face while I'm recovering from this sudden, terrifying, yet curable illness. It is difficult to put into words how genuinely thankful we are. We are blessed to have people in our lives that are so loving, encouraging, and kind. It is because of your encouragement and support that we are fighting this with such strength and determination.

Thank you again, from the bottom of our hearts.
Joe, Jenn, and John Venegas

Then and now and next
Apr 8, 2014

A little re-cap.

After months of seemingly random symptoms (lack of energy, cloudy thinking, nausea, dizziness, trouble breathing, infections, headaches, unexplainable bruising, to name a few), I was diagnosed with Acute Lymphoblastic Leukemia, with the Philadelphia + chromosome, in January. Leukemia is a blood disease, is chromosomal (my genes decided to do their own thing and my immune system didn't correct it), and is unheard of for a female in her 40's. What I have is extremely rare - of course it is. I was immediately admitted and have since been in and out of the hospital for extended stays and 3 chemo treatments. I have also been in remission (no apparent cancer cells) since my first chemo treatment, but the only "sure thing" for long term remission is a bone marrow or stem cell transplant. The transplant would give me a new immune system that will identify the cancer as alien and destroy it, unlike my current broken immune system that would identify cancer as family and let it back in. I have responded amazingly well to the treatments so far and have surprised the docs at every level.

Luckily, my sister Becky has been tested and is a perfect match, making her my stem cell donor. This is a miracle (there's a 25% chance of one of my siblings being a match) and she's going through a lot of pain and sacrifice to make this possible. The doctors call her my "twin" as she and I are a perfect match. This is wonderful because that means there is a reduced chance of her cells rejecting me as their new home. I'll look very familiar to them!

So now what...

I'm off to the hospital where they'll do the stem cell transplant on Friday to start the next stage of my adventure. Although I've done chemo before, this is entirely different and I have no idea what to expect. It's 2 days of a high dose chemo followed by 4 days of high dose radiation, twice a day. On the 17th, they will "harvest" an unbelievable amount of stem cells from Becky and transfuse them (through an IV type line) into me. This is all new and unpredictable and scary and exciting. I'll be in the hospital for 3-5 weeks and

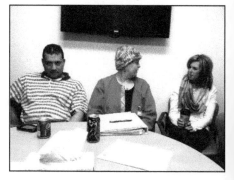

under strict supervision and guidelines. Like before, all visitors, if any, will have to not only wear the mask, but a gown and cap as well. I won't even be able to see John. Boo. All for my health and best chance of recovery.

Once they see my numbers are recovering, I'll be discharged to the next stage - 30 days at an extended stay facility nearby. I will need a caregiver 24/7 and as sterile an environment as possible. The packet addressing guidelines and restrictions on diet and food prep alone is 20 pages long. The duties and responsibilities of the caregiver is also extensive, and I don't envy any of them. Thankfully I have an amazing support system with my family and they have graciously volunteered whatever time necessary to make sure I'm comfortable and have the best chance at a full recovery.

My recovery is called "the 100 days" and starts on the 17th - day "zero" is always the first day of transplant. The goal is to get me back to my normal life as soon as possible, but the road to get there is tedious. The first 30 days in the hospital, the next 30 days at the extended stay facility, then home for 30-40 days. I'll have tests and clinic visits 3 times a week to monitor my recovery. My restrictions will slowly be eased and I'll be able to do normal things like drive, eat out, and shop - hopefully - that's our combined goal. Maybe even get back to work part-time. That's MY goal. However, the doctor team was very clear in letting me know recovery could take up to a year or more before I feel like myself again. That also means the restrictions are in place until then as well. I'll have to replace many of my favorite things (gardening, camping, being outdoors, etc.) with less dangerous indoor ones. UGH.

But there could be complications along the way. Graft Versus Host Disease (GVHD) is the most common and involves a reverse rejection by Becky's stem cells. It's common for the new cells to attack my bone marrow and other organs because they are foreign (not Becky's) and this could be bad. And good. A little is ok, a lot is not. I could also get any number of infections from bacteria, mold, spores, viruses and any number of both common and uncommon ailments. It's a very scary thing as it can't be predicted and these "complications" are very risky as I don't have an immune system.

Sooooo...I am aware this update is rather clinical and less personal. I've been reflecting, remembering, and purging a lot of information lately, which feels good going into this next phase. I'm glad it'll be a new facility, new staff, new routines, and new treatment. I'm also glad there will be some similarities - hospital room and bed, checking vitals, vocabulary, pajamas, taking meds, answering the same monotonous questions, being monitored all the time for every possible physical change. And spending precious time with each of my family members creating special memories, laughing, crying, and eating Voodoo Donuts! Lol.

I think I'm ready...

Tammy - *I'm sending prayers every step of the way. I know you and I were not close friends in school, but you are a true inspiration and I am honored to watch you go through this through caring bridge and Facebook. You are blessed with an amazing support system and spirit. I pray for you and those with you and cry at your updates. Thank you for keeping us updated on your progress.*

Janet - *Hey Jenn. I just read your message, and I am just bowled over with all of the stages to your new recovery. I think about you all the time and send love and strength to get through this. With your positive attitude and fortitude, I'm sure this will be a success. Lots of love to all of you, especially you and Becky. Love Janet*

Steph - *You are ready. You are. You've got this, Jenny.*

Robert - *Jenn, life has always been full of challenges and surprises. reading your blogs says that you are ready for whatever comes your way. I will put you on our prayer list at church. You and Becky are in our prayers. Love, LeRoy and Barb*

Robert - *Jenn, our prayers are sent out to you and Becky during your coming challenges. We will place you on our Church prayer list. LeRoy and Barb*

Mary - *You can take the teacher out of the school, but the teacher still remains. I have learned so much about your illness through reading about your journey Jenn. Every journey is different and one remarkable thing stands out to me as I read yours. You are a resilient and positive person and you face these incredible challenges head-on.*

You are going to get through these 100 days and your body will become strong again. I hold you up in my prayers and I hope you know that we miss you at the high school and that we will see you there next school year!

cas - *Good luck, Mama V! I know you'll be strong and have as quick and easy of a recovery as possible! You and your family are in my prayers!*

Chapter 4

Breakdowns, Detours,

and Roadblocks

Rough Doesn't Begin to Explain it
Apr 15, 2014

I thought I had been through the first stages of chemo and "flown" through them. And I suppose I did. And I thought I knew what nausea, and muscle and joint pain were, and diarrhea, and headaches, and all the other side-effects were like...until now. What I went through was a fairy tale of symptoms that could have been up there with flying a kite or going to the circus. This new state of reality is agonizing. Whatever you've heard about chemo being terrible is true and worse. The pain, and tears, and discomfort, and feeling like the only way to help is to go to sleep but you can't do that because it hurts so much. And Radiation is the DEVIL. You sit in a plexi-glass box with your hands on your lap 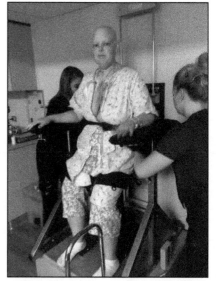 and rice bags taped between your knees and on your feet while a beam of radiation is directed at you from both sides like a projector or flashlight. Except it's the most exhausting thing ever and makes you feel humiliated. THEN day 3-4 of radiation you sit on the most uncomfortable bicycle seat ever, again while they blast poison at your system. And the contraption looks like something the Little Rascals made -

with plyboard and 2 by 4's and pulleys to get the height right. I was on a soap box while radiation killed everything in me. I'm glad that part is over, but now we wait for the outcomes. Chemo made my hair fall out - an outward sign. Radiation is a whole different animal and the thing that sucks is that all my reactions are behind by about a week. So I won't know the full gravity of high dose radiation or chemo until after the stem cell transplant. And won't know how I react to the stem cells until closer to the end of April, about 10 days from now. This is the hardest thing I've ever had to do. They say it's like a third-degree sunburn from the inside out.

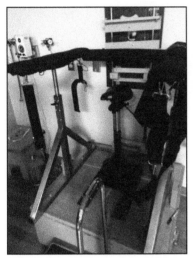

And I'm not ready to talk about the stem cell transplant that took place Thursday yet. It's impossibly hard to comprehend all that is happening to me and it's all surreal. I feel like the past 3 months has been about whatever is killing me and treatments to do so. The day of the transplant turned the corner, climbed the summit, was a momentum changer, or however you want to describe it. I went from dying to living. But I feel my body is dying more than living.

My blessings remain my sister and my family. Without them I wouldn't be looking at much of a future and they make all the little things stay little and keep me focused on the big picture.

Rex - _I can't fathom the physical & mental pain, misery suffering you are going through right now...my only barometer is the pain, misery & suffering that Jesus Christ must've had while dying on the cross for all of us. He must've felt completely humiliated, embarrassed & hopeless as he was exposed before friends & foe on a wooden cross ... ultimately to his death. Jenn, my hope & prayers now are for the horrible effects of the radiation to subside & ultimately go away! I know I can't fix this problem for you (which frustrates the hell out of me) but I can ask God Almighty to have mercy on you & help ease your pain ok? God bless you honey. I love you always...now & forever, DAD_

Valerie - I wish i could put my arms around you! Without hurting you. <3

Julie - There are no words...I can only offer my prayers.

Gail - we Care So Much And Can't Begin To Imagine What You Are Going Through. Your Story Has Truly Touched Us And We Will Continue To Pray. Love Gail And Jack

Kathy - I am so still praying for you! Your name is at my computer on my desk and I pray.

Mary - The old adage that it is always darkest before the dawn is a true one. I am sorry that you are in this living hell and believe that it will be worth it Jenn. I know you do too.

The family:
Apr 17, 2014 (Good Friday)

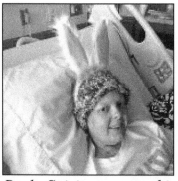

It's here! *The bone marrow just arrived at Jenny's room! Due to Becky's bravery and patience, the lab was able to collect all the stem cells needed to fuel Jennifer with new life today. Thanks Becky! It has been a long, long day to get to this happy moment; Jenn weathered two long rounds of radiation to ruin the rest of the enemy cells. Now she is ready to take on the new healthy stuff donated by Beck. Spirits are very high now. Mom, dad and I are with Jenn, and Ryan, Becky, Joe and John are on the way. In a short while, we are going to pray and share thanks for this miracle. How in the world can one person give their blood, their heart, to save another? Jesus showed the way, and Becky has taken His example seriously. What a day for Jenn to receive new life!! There really are no words for how amazing this is.... we all feel blessed beyond belief!*

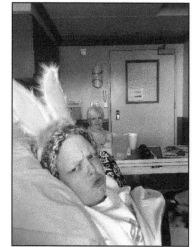

This is my MAD face. And I love Mom's photo bomb in the back!

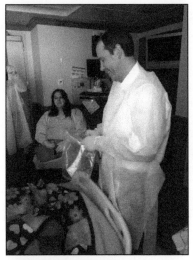

The Doctor held the stem cells with such reverence, as though it was my life in his hands. It was and he completely understood the weight of these moments. And Becky in the background so freely volunteering to suffer for me. I am forever grateful.

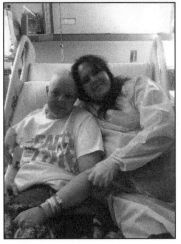

Now we are truly twins!

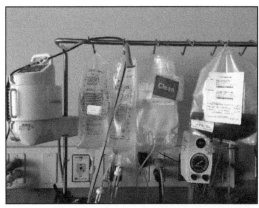

My cocktail

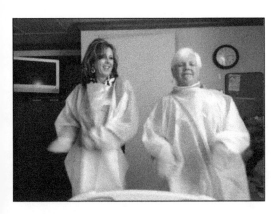

The HAPPY dance!

Can you believe this archaic looking thing was responsible for keeping me alive?

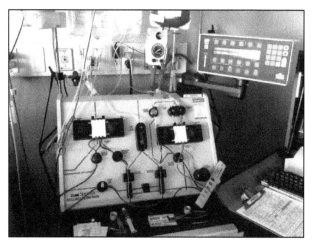

Mom, Dad, Becky, and Steph. I'm the one in the middle with the bald head.

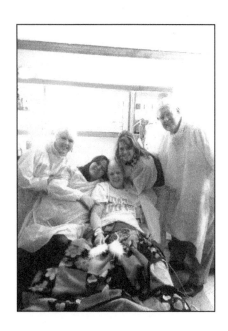

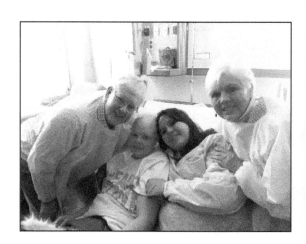

Becky donating her stem cells after an agonizing week of her own treatments. They had to boost her stem cells with a medication that made her bones, muscles, and joint scream with pain. She was a trooper though. Happy to do it. She's my angel.

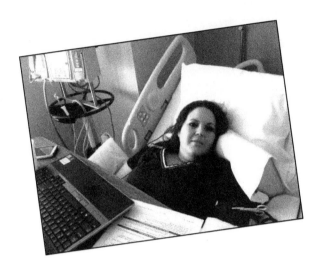

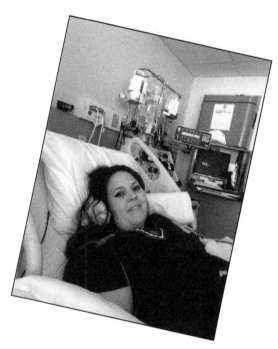

The next two weeks of entries are based on memories, reading my hand written journals from during those days, and conversations I've had with people since then. These two weeks were by far the worst thing I've ever been through and was in no condition to write, or communicate at the time for that matter. I added these journals/memories and pictures because it is very important to me to write my whole story so that others, patients, caregivers, and staff, can have a realistic understanding of the purely horrific, yet survivable, situations the human body and spirit can endure.

The Week I Never Saw Coming
April 18, 2014

This week I am dying. Literally. And I'm writing this from the journals me and my family kept while I was here because I was incapacitated from the Chemo, Radiation, and my cells dying and there was no way I could have updated my journal during this time.

It started with the stomach and guts in agonizing cramps and uncontrollable diarrhea. This was amplified by the pain medications that left me slow and unaware of much. I had a portable commode right next to my bed and there were times I still didn't make it in time. It was like my body was leaking out of me. And from what I'm told, that was exactly what was happening. The purpose of the treatments was to kill ALL my bone marrow and stem cells so the new healthy ones would have a room to move into. The dying cells were sluffing off all at once and there was a fear of other complications related to this. Thankfully that didn't happen, but my body was dying none the less. Consider this the "all we can do is watch, wait, and control the symptoms" approach because everyone reacts differently to the treatments. This is where it became even more apparent that cancer affects everyone differently. I guess you could say you are the owner of your own personal cancer to include treatments, side effects, medications, reactions, and recovery. I was in agony, and didn't even know it.

I Can Feel Everything and I'm in Agony
April 19, 2014

I woke up this morning and my tongue was so swollen I could hardly breathe. My mouth and throat were on fire. Turning grey and dying with blisters. My whole body hurts. Feet, hands, headache from hell. My back. I couldn't find a comfortable position but was too tired to move, but my body was trembling none the less. I'm cold, then on fire. My toes and fingers sting from neuropathy (numbness). I know that sounds crazy, but picture putting your hands in a bucket of ice for 10 minutes, then pulling them out. IT STINGS. Zaps of pain like no other.

I can't swallow so I'm not eating or drinking, at all. Can't swallow pills so my medicine pole looks like a Christmas tree and they had to put an additional monitor on my pole. I started throwing up in the afternoon, but all that came up was water and my pills. Talk about the worst possible scenario. Not only can I not swallow going down because of the pain, now it's coming up like acid and it's even worse.

I can literally feel every cell in my body and they're all pissed off. And fighting against death and me and my body. And I have no defense other than blindly just going through every minute as they come. What else can I do? There isn't a moment of peace between the pain, shaking, spasms, and treatments. I felt like I was watching a movie of someone else going through it. Absolutely surreal. If you haven't had chemo or radiation, I'm not sure you fully understand what surreal really means. This is hell.

Easter
April 20, 2014

I didn't sleep at all last night from the constant cramps and diarrhea. My jaw, mouth, and throat are on fire and I can hardly breathe it hurts so much. They've put me on a pain killer, but it doesn't seem to be working. I also have a suction tube (like the one at the dentists) I can use to drain the mucus and saliva from my mouth rather than swallowing it, but it isn't giving me any relief. The pain meds gave me uncontrollable and painful arm and leg spasms so they finally gave me a self-administered morphine drip. Here's where the craziness started.

I couldn't recognize anyone. I called my sister-in-law my donor, which she wasn't, and probably could have been declared insane. I was in and out of consciousness. I remember thinking, "just get this cup to your mouth…" and then waking up with my water spilled all over me because I had lost consciousness somewhere between the tray 18 inches away from me and my mouth. This happened with everything. I forgot I had to go to the bathroom. Couldn't remember what day it was. It was painful for my family to watch. At first it was funny to see me in and out, passing out right in the middle of a conversation and waking up finishing the sentence. But then it wasn't. John came one time and wouldn't come back because he couldn't see his mom in that condition. I don't blame him. But how heart wrenching is that?

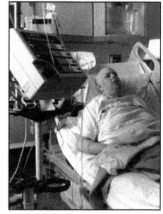

Visitors
April 21, 2014

Today was very strange. In addition to my normal doctor and nurse visitors, I had several other visitors, some real and some not-so-real. My mom came with clean laundry, peppermint for my tummy, and lots of laughter. I wrote in my journal, "I LOVE her and her visits. It's what I'm fighting for." That was real. I had a visit from the "Art Lady" who came once a week to help patients find methods of stress management and coping through different art activities. Coloring books, water colors, origami, "I Am" drawings and that sort of thing. It was nice to take my mind off things for a while. I can only image how she felt though when I would suddenly be asleep in the middle of a paint stroke. I'd wake up and continue like it didn't happen. I wish someone had taken video. This was also real.

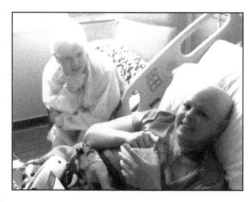

But today I started hallucinating. I remember them well and they were hilarious. Not even a bit concerning. The White Rabbit from Alice in Wonderland was playing hide and seek behind the television and in the bathroom door. Sometimes he'd sneak under my bed. The furniture had a life of its own and would occasionally "bend" and then pop back into shape. There were all kinds of little animals and creatures running all over my room. It kinda reminded me of Bambi or a fairy forest or something. It was nice to be so distracted by these visitors, I have to admit. Being in a different world was a wonderful escape. These visitors were not real. It's funny to note that in my journal this entry was labeled "other random side effects". I find this hilarious.

Reflections
April 22 – 26, 2014

The rest of this week was a complete blur. Literally in and out of consciousness, hitting my morphine button because of the pain, and loss of time completely. I had the worst case of Mucositis (mouth sores, swelling, pain) the doctors had ever seen. They were worried that if my mouth and throat got any more swollen I wouldn't be able to breathe and they'd have to put me on a ventilator. It was touch and go for days. I was using mouth washes to the best of my ability that were temporarily soothing, but even ice chips were too much for my mouth to handle.

By the end of the week though, around Saturday, I started healing and feeling better physically – no more concern about a ventilator - but very sad and depressed emotionally. They said this was normal but I didn't like it. It made me moody, grumpy, short-tempered, and I wasn't a very nice person.

The Port Fiasco
April 28, 2014

When I first checked in, the first procedure they did was surgically install a Port (direct line) to accommodate all the treatments and to alleviate being poked all over. It's located in my upper chest and is supposed to heal right into my skin and create a protected seal that would allow me to take showers, go swimming, and otherwise lead a normal life. However, from the get-go, it never looked like it was healing to me. There was one side that never really formed a scab or connected to the tube, and I told the nurses repeatedly of my concern. So did my parents and sibs. The nurses weren't worried at all. In addition, they said I would be able to take the dressing off in a day or two and I'd be fine. This terrified me, I told them this, but again they said I had nothing to worry about. Well, guess what? The very night they took off the dressing, I rolled over in bed and out popped my tube…AND ALL MY NEW STEM CELLS. NO JOKE. They were pouring out of my chest and I was screaming while placing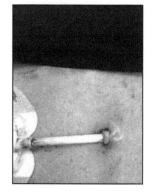

my palm over the hole. It was gushing. GUSHING. Of course it was because it was directly connected to a major artery and it was evacuating through the hole at massive speed. I was covered head to toe in blood. It was pooling up on the bed and on the floor and I was in hysterics. The first nurse that came in the room was brazen enough to ask me why I pulled it out. I would have launched myself at her had I not been more concerned about holding my life in my hands. THE BITCH! I – we – had told them for days it was going to happen, and it did, and they blamed me? What? Get this straight, it was surgically inserted into my aorta for the specific purpose of

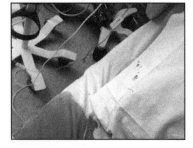 being embedded and UNREMOVABLE, and just pulling out would have been so painful I would have passed out. But what did I know, right? I've had treatments, was weak, on pain meds, barely coherent, affected by Chemo brain, and had the steady hand (which was impossible) to just pull it out? During this time I was also shivering and shaking so badly I couldn't hold a cup or take my medications on my own.

So the first nurse couldn't handle the scene and called in all her resources. I then had 2-3 nurses asking me why I pulled it out. The funniest thing, if you can call it funny, was when the 2nd nurse asked me to move my hand and the blood spurted all over her face, chest, and bed. She gasped and left the room. I was actually in more control than they were, holding my hand to my chest and screaming orders. Not letting them touch it unless they had a plan to stop the bleeding and the tragic loss of all the stem cells so painfully and carefully harvested, donated by my sister, leaving my body. Is this happening? I even had the clarity to take pictures of the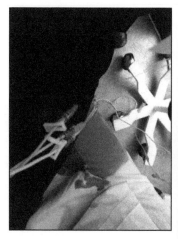

mess. Thank goodness I did because I could show the doctors what had really happened, and not the version the nurses were going to tell. Which they did.

I have to do what????
May 2, 2014

Each day has had a very individualistic theme to it and thank goodness my memory sucks or I'd probably have flown the coop by now. From now on I'm going to name the days I'm having because each day is so hard to remember and has such personality of its own.

This is your brain on drugs...

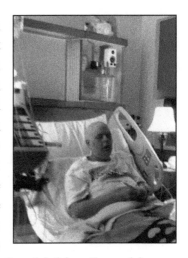

Today I woke up from a drug induced stupor at 11:00 am (I feel like I'm in college all over again - except last night was NO fun at all!). I am having a detox-like reaction from one of the drugs the pain medications I was put on over the past week to control the torturous mouth and throat sores and complications (can't swallow, can't drink so you know you can't swallow either, and when you do have to swallow, the pain is excruciating) associated with it. Radiation shares so willingly. However, I got to use the awesome machine that had that cool little self-serve button I could click if I wanted another short dose now: you know, one of those things you've always wanted to try, but you never get a chance to. Anyway, I know you're thinking I used it too much and you'd be wrong. I used less than a quarter of the allotted dose and was doing so they could take me off the med. I'm thinking, "Great! Less to lug around with the IV pole (I named him Phil (he "fills" me up)." Then came the nighttime. I think I was most upset because I called it days ago and they didn't believe me. "Do you think I could be allergic to something? " NAH was the answer so they started me on the poison anyway. Within minutes I was so itchy I thought I was going to scratch my skin off. I began having horrible tremors and shakes. I'm now on a recovery dose off of the morphine. I'm so antsy I get terrible shakes and even writing is hell which is why I'm using a recorder to get this narrated instead of writing it because I don't have the patience to sit still or even type. It's like restless leg syndrome amplified and scary. So I'm going nighty night. And hopefully won't have to let you know until tomorrow about how I'm doing.

Rex - Hang in there Jenn - You will be just fine. It makes sad that your recovery is still so painful but, hopefully, you'll be able to leave the hospital real soon & feel so much better! Love ya lots, DAD

Mary - Even with what you are going through, you keep that sense of humor! "Phil" cracked me up. I must say, I do remember some mornings in college when I woke up pretty shaky and sick. But had fun memories of the night before! I like the idea of your naming each day because it takes a life of its own. Five years from now when you think about this period of your life, maybe it will seem like one long night in retrospect. In so many ways, you have been your own best advocate Jenn. By paying attention to your body, you got diagnosed early. By paying attention to what the meds were doing to you, you got weaned off before they made you even sicker.Hang in there and remember how many people are rooting you on.

Jennifer - That means so much to me coming from a person like you, Mary. I have a hard time remembering this morning let alone a week ago, so writing makes it better. I also have a short journal of my meds and times, reactions or non, and general feelings when appropriate. I thought it was silly at first, until the gave me something I was allergic to, and once doubled a dose, and what's worked in the past and why/not. I had a nurse ask me last week, "Jenn, what's your journal say?" Too funny. But thank you for validating it is necessary and helpful and who I am. That means the most, that you know who I am and can probably visualize me at the window typing. Much Love, Jenn

Introductions are Necessary
May 3, 2014

My first stay at the hospital started some interesting things that never really got left behind. For instance, I had to be hooked by IV (it was a PICC line - to be continued) to one of those medical poles holding a bag of something attached to this cord of something (I mean really, how much saline does one person need) that is supposed to be doing something. Meds - pain, anti-fungal, antiviral, anti-diarrheal, anti-bacterial, anti-histamine, anti-nausea, etc... I had to roll that damn thing with me everywhere. It was a part of me, my shadow, and I was tired of it. To the bathroom, shower (he stayed his distance outside the curtain), walking the halls, and to the doctors right across the way. So one day I called him 'Phil'. It just came out from nowhere. "Come on Phil, let's go to the bathroom." And there it stands. We have decorated Phil with Bronco stuff (didn't 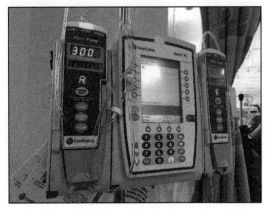 help), Valentines stuff, hats and scarves, and most recently we called him "Badd Ass" - because Phil can hold technically 8 bags of stuff and I had 12 going. Ridiculous. And most recently he became Lucy's tree because he's bear with only one bag of stuff that I take for an hour twice a day. Now I'll have to take a version of Phil to my next destination (extended stay near the hospital) for routine treatments we'll have to do. We're looking for names for the new Phil so let me know if you have any suggestions.

I can't go on without mentioning the bane to my existence, El Diablo. This little pain in the ass (PITA) nicely measures and dole s out the appropriate amount of medication you should be getting, but also monitors air in the lines, kinks or "Occlusions", and when treatments are done. Then it beeps. And beeps and beeps and beeps. And it doesn't care what time it is or what you're doing; it demands immediate assistance. And then you have to call the nurse, which could take MANY minutes, before she can come in and straighten your line or flick the bubbles or just turn it off. And sometimes ED waits until the nurse just leaves the room and busts out with another blast of beeps. And you can hear everyone else's beeps too. Like a crooked symphonic torture. I have strong dislike for El Diablo, but he's just doing his job. I just wish he didn't do it so well.

The next character in our story is 'Flow'. Can you guess? She's the new-fangled vitals machine that measures everything going on in your body through blood pressure, CO_2 readings, heart rates, temperature and on. She also has the tightest grasp of ANYONE I've ever met. Wrestlers, Mechanics, Gator Hunters, Nascar Racers, and Oil Riggers, have NOTHING ON HER. Her cuff of varying sizes can apparently be placed in different locations like the ankle or wrist if they can't use arms (like I couldn't for a while). And then the torture begins. The first time (if you're doing it in a series like I did) the cuff inflates (engages) to something past what it "thinks" you'll measure out, usually over 160 (that's the top number in your blood pressure, 160 over something, normally 120/80). I was lucky to get my dad's system and have low blood pressure (110-75), but Flow didn't care. She just kept a pumping until my arm nearly exploded. No joke - my hand was so red and getting so swollen I was afraid I'd be spurting blood from my fingertips any minute. And changing colors like a chameleon; red, purple, grey. Then the sound you've been waiting for, silence happens and you hope she starts doing her thing, but no. You have to wait for her to slowly make up her mind to start counting and slowly - and I mean SLOWLY - let the air out. It. Was. Torture. And some days I had to do that on a schedule every 15 or 30 minutes, and you can be sure Flow was never late. Oh no. you'd hear the pump and cringe knowing what is coming next. And then there's the CO2 monitor thingy they put on your finger and they want the reading to stay over 90. Well the whole darn floor erupts with sirens when you happen to dip to 89 so don't ever let that happen. They also make you wear oxygen if it ever drops below 90; just take my advice and make sure you breathe deeply and keep your blood oxygenated. (Do a few easy and slow jumping jacks before your next appointment. It'll help the CO2 and won't necessarily raise the blood pressure...so I'm told).

Last but not least, is Chicky (named after the PICC Chicks). She's my PICC line that connects through a vein in my upper arm and has three "lumens" (the little fingers that connect to the IV). She's awesome and has treated me well. We use her to both infuse medications and draw blood without having to prick my skin every time. We all had to learn how to flush her and look for a blood return, but that's easy. She's your friend.

Can't forget the Nurses. Period. They do everything and get no credit for it. They know medications and interactions better than the Docs themselves. They change sheets in all conditions, throw away trash, get water and ice, hook up and monitor the IV lines, and literally save lives. They did for me last week and I can't thank them enough! They are called Angels.

Rex - You make be hooked to an IV pole sound like a real fun adventure! Just kidding...It would drive me nuts. The name "PHIL" for "fill-er-up" seems very appropriate honey. At this time, I think I'd call it the "SHADOW" or something we can't say on Caring Bridge!!!!! We all look forward to the next phase of your journey ... Getting out of the hospital & moving into your new digs! Onward & upwards ...

It's On!!
May 4, 2014

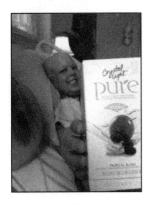

I just heard that a lady down the hall that came in about the same time I did, about my age, with the same diagnosis and treatment plan, is getting ready to leave sometime this week. If you know me at all....IT'S ON! Let's do this!

I'll eat whatever slime covered crap you give me. I'll walk 1000 miles down this ridiculous 80-foot corridor. I'll take any stupid medicine and endure any side effect to get out of here.

BRING IT!!!

Tomorrow!
May 6, 2014

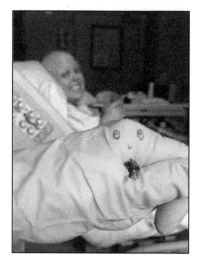

Yep! I'm getting out tomorrow! And on to the next stage of recovery. They call it the 100 days and technically I'm on day 19. For the next 4 weeks I'll be moving to a residence home to slowly transition, with most of the same restrictions in place, to home. During my stay at the residence home, I'll be able to go home on weekends, and the whole plan is to "transition" (I know, that word is used a lot), back to my normal life by the end of the 100 days. I'll still have to go to the clinic 3 days a week to get lab work done with that tapering off by the end. That doesn't mean I'll be back to top shape, but I'll be able to drive and go shopping, and garden, and camp, and ride my dirt bike, and be a mom and wife, and restore all the activities, at a limited pace, I have always enjoyed. Hopefully, that also includes going back to work part time this fall, but I'm in no hurry. I want to make sure this thing has been CURED; not in remission, not at bay, not healed. CURED. I'll never have to be afraid of it again. Isn't that an amazing thought? I can't quite wrap my head around it yet; the whole cancer thing is still rather a blur. But moving on is always a good thing. And I'm ready. After fur hospital stays, two of them 25 days or longer, I'm ready for home. And hopefully this whole experience, with the exception of the things I've learned (who my friends are, the incredible blessings in my life, how to "be" and take things one day at a time, how to let things go) will be a flash of a memory by this time next year and we'll be celebrating my "new" birthday on April 17th, 2015!!

Gina - This makes my heart happy. Such a good road to be travelling. Yay you!
Amy - Such great news. I keep saying you are an inspiration to all of us following you on this difficult journey, and you've even been able to keep a sense of humor. Thank you for being so real. I'll continue to be praying.
Jim - Yay Jenn!! So happy to hear you progressing through these healing steps! Love the positivity-SO healthy! You are THE BOMB girl! You're an inspiration!
Rex - We're all ready for your new digs ... Change of pace, change of view & change of attitude! From now on called it's called "RECOVERY" ;-) Love ya, Dad
Valerie - I'm so excited for you Jenn!! Way to fight! Congratulations!
Mary - HAPPY DANCE!!!!!

Kathy - *I'm sooo happy for you!!!! I will continue to pray for you as the transition progresses. And, I will pray for you to quickly regain your strength and feel better than you did before this ever started. You have been an inspiration to me and such a blessing. You will never know how much your experience has touched my life. Keep on Keeping on - there is a light at the end of this tunnel and He is shining brightly through you!*

Jeana - *I can't wait to be celebrating with you next April on your new birthday :). Right around the time for our next AVID spring celebration (which will go much smoother when I have you back to help me, lol :). So happy to hear that you are truly on the way back!!!!*

Chapter 5

Coasting

Day 27
May 14, 2014

I am 27 days past my stem cell transplant, at the residence home, and doing AMAZING!! I have enjoyed every bit of my return to humanity and every new normal thing. Things like fresh air; I cried when it rained, and I could smell the new air. Touching the snow instead of just watching it fall. Using a full-sized shower towel. Not having to watch out for tubing and IV lines. Being able 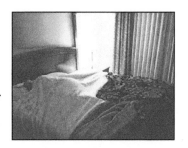 to stand up and go anywhere I wanted without boundaries or attached to anything. Shopping and being able to pick out the things I want instead of making a list for someone else. Eating real food. Being able to relax for hours at a time knowing no one would come in and disturb me. Start a project more than 5 minutes long without the fear of being interrupted. Wear real clothes and put earrings back on (my special joy was that my nose ring hole didn't heal up and I can still wear one...weird I know). The little things we all take for granted, including me, are daily and valued and priceless.

I'm still not out of the woods until day 100, so even though I'm experiencing a lot of freedoms I didn't have at the hospital, I still must have a caregiver with me 24 hours a day, 7 days a week. It's part of the transition. They flush my PICC line so it doesn't clot shut or get infected, help me with meals, sleep here, take me to my appointments three times a week, and keep an eye on my side effects like fever, rashes, pain, etc. This has been so hard on them. The whole experience. Gracefully giving up time during the week to be with me. Scheduling who would be with me when. Meals. They're having to take care of my like I was an infant, which technically I am. I was born again April 17 and I'm less than a month old. I'm just a quick learner and can walk, talk, and eat solid food. However, I also throw up, have diarrhea, no hair, and limited vision, just like a baby would. But spending time with my family members, individually, has been priceless and I've treasured and been present for every moment. I might not remember them all with this chemo brain and all, but I know I've laughed and cried a lot and had terrific conversations that are dear to me.

My counts are all going in the right direction and I'm seeing improvements in my energy, appetite, activity level, attitude, and sleep. Every day I am getting better and looking forward a little more. Since my diagnosis in January I have learned patience and to take one day at a time. The future is undetermined and can change at any moment. I have learned how to just "be". Gracefully, authentically, and emotionally, I feel more and more present every day. It was harder in the hospital because I didn't want to be there, and the meds didn't let me.

Looking forward, I know that I'll go home full time early in June and be around day 50; half way there. The one thing preventing me from a sooner-than-later recovery would be complications related to the transplant. Things like infections, organ function, and any internal issue ("gut") could postpone my return to normal. I don't want that so I still have to be cautious and use common sense when it comes to being around people and what I eat.

So all things considered and counted, day 100 will land late in July and life will be back to "normal", best case scenario. So pray for no complications and a swift and complete recovery! In the meantime, I'll be walking stairs and using the weights to get my strength back!

Rex - Honey - After just having been w/ u ... I can't express how thrilled I am to see the huge progress being made each day now after the miraculous bone marrow transplant w/ Becky a few weeks ago! Just being you while having breakfast today actually SITTING UP was amazing after watching you lying in bed all tied up to an IV pole for the past 4 months. Let's pray now that the worst is behind you & now we can focus on a full recovery no matter how long that may take! Bring it on...Love ya, DAD

Take me with you!
May 15, 2014

I have a long summer of very restricted indoor activities in my immediate future as I transition back to my life and will have to miss MANY fun times along the way. Since the benefit in March, it has been a priceless gift to me when my friends have taken the orange koozie with them to their adventures and send pictures of them to me. It gets me out of my room, if even for a moment, and makes me feel like I'm right there with them enjoying the event or just the time together. It's therapeutic, and happy, and thoughtful. I've been to the Rockies Home Opener, the Avalanche Playoffs (boo), New York, and MANY restaurants and such along the way (there are some posted on this site already). SO... please consider taking your koozie to your next event, meal, activity, party, trip, etc. and take a picture with it for me. Post on here, or Facebook, or text it to me, but please... take me with you!!

Gina - I want a koozie to take along with me!! Where can I get one?
Michelle - You are going to have a fabulous summer full of love, happiness, health and adventure!!! xoxo
Rex - Jenn - You're with me wherever I go & whatever I'm doing! Love ya, DAD
Mitch - Jennifer, we pray for you daily. I so no matter where we go you are always with us.

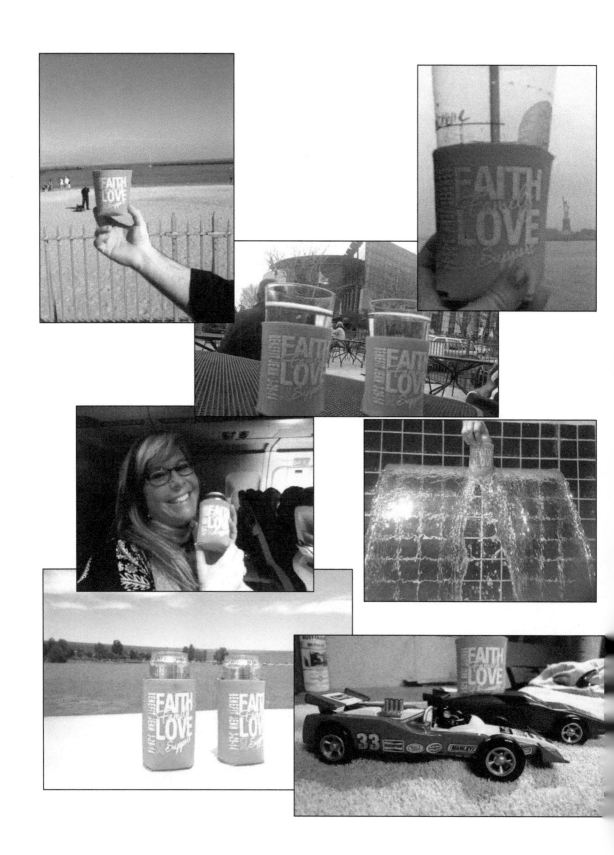

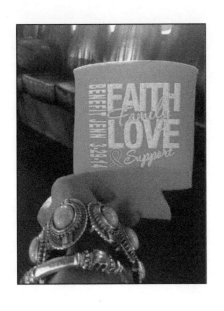

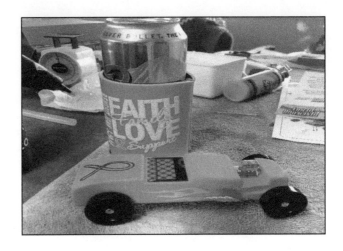

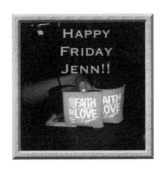

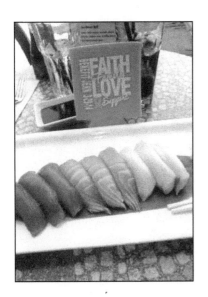

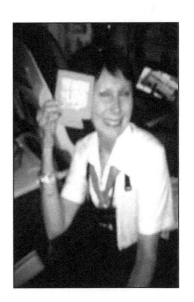

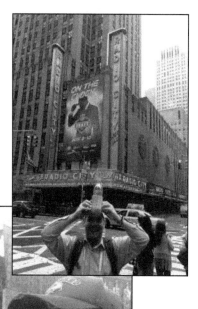

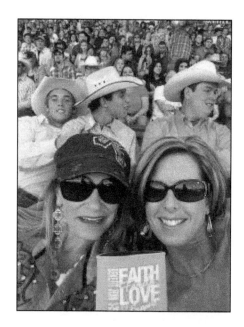

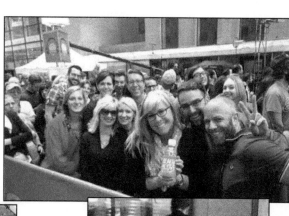

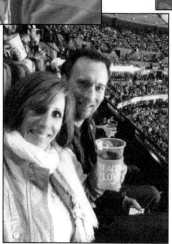

Day 45
Jun 1, 2014

So I've been at an apartment suite facility since I got out of the hospital on Day 20, and it's amazing how the days just pass by. I'm already at day 45 and almost halfway through the prescribed 100-day recovery time!! You'd think I have lots of down time, and relatively speaking I suppose I do, but my time still passes so quickly. The staff here have been AMAZINGLY ACCOMMODATING every step of the way. Since the minute I checked in and they gave me a room upgrade, to the numerous times they've generously gone above and beyond, even coming to the room at 8:30pm to fix our DVD player, they have been gracious and giving.

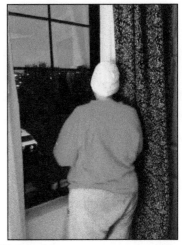

My one-bedroom suite includes a bedroom for me, a full kitchen so we can cook "sanitarily", TV's in both the bedroom and the main room, a hideaway bed for my visitors, and all the other normal amenities hotels usually provide. They also have daily morning breakfast buffet and an afternoon "social hour" where they serve free dinner and cocktails: a personal favorite for my caregivers on Tuesday, Wednesday, and Thursday evenings! It has a pool, hot tub, laundry, workout area, professional area (office with computers and fax, etc.), provides shuttle rides to all my appointments, and a pantry for last minute items and snacks. I mention these things because I feel that although all these things are wonderful, I can only enjoy some of them.

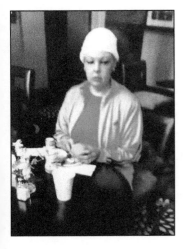

I can't eat most of the items on the buffets, unless they're individually wrapped (like a muffin), because of the potential for the spreading of germs and disease. I can't eat the eggs, bacon, waffles, fruit bar, pastries, or anything else with a spoon or serving utensil that others have shared. I can't have the wings, hot dogs or hamburgers, or salads they provide in the afternoon. I have become a genuine germaphobe and carry Purell with me everywhere I go. I can have an occasional glass of wine and enjoy the company of my guests on the patio in the back. It has many comfortable seating arrangements, a fire pit, and access to the basketball court and pool areas. It's very nice and I love the time outside, but it's different from the normal everyone else is experiencing. I can't use the pool or hot tub because they are known to be germ nests, and my infantile immune system can't fight off all the cooties that might be floating around. As free as I feel, I am still faced with many restrictions. I can open windows as I please, take showers when I want to, walk to the main desk without being chaperoned, but I couldn't drive until last Friday when I finally got the go-ahead. Shopping is possible, but I wear a mask and can only go in short bits of time because my endurance needs some work. I can go outside but can't be in the sun and have to wear sunscreen (another common-sense thing). And for the most part, I still have a caregiver with me 100% of the time to help with things like flushing my lines (which my mom is horrified of doing), and meals, and assisting the visiting nurse with infusions.

I look back to the day I arrived here, without a voice due to the radiation, unable to touch my toes having lost all flexibility, having trouble with stairs because my legs forgot how to do them and had lost their strength, unable to eat more than a few mouthfuls of anything, needing help standing up because my balance was on vacation, and wondering if I could make it down the long hall to my room. After three weeks I have realized how much I've improved having a voice again, doing many flights of stairs and the halls aren't an issue, my flexibility and strength are returning, my appetite is back and foods are tasting more 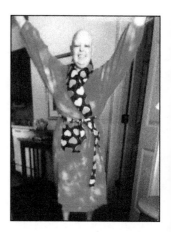 normal again, and I'm losing some of the things holding me back. I've been cleared to drive, have taken a turn in my meds and am taking many less that treat side-effects, and a few more that show signs of improvement - I'm into the maintenance stage and that's a wonderful thing. Oh yeah - my hair is growing back!! Slowly, but a great sign of my improving health!

Because the radiation and chemo removed most of my immune system, that also means it destroyed all the immunities I had built up either through exposure or through the shots we begin taking as infants. I am no longer immune to Measles, Mumps, Rubella, Chicken Pox, Polio and anything else I received a shot for through the past 42 years. And I won't be re-immunized for a year from transplant...next spring. Talk about walking through life with fear. It's good to know that most people these days have also been immunized so the chances are slim of me catching anything...but the chances are still there and pose the most danger to a full recovery - also called "complications".

And still there are so many things to look forward to. I've been cleared to return to work in the fall. I can be a chauffeur for John and his friends again. I'm cooking a little, doing some laundry, helping with the daily stuff at home, going on short shopping trips, but still using a tremendous amount of common sense (washing hands, not digging in the dirt, being careful around others and wearing a mask). It's all leading to a complete remission and a normal life again. Next Friday will be my last day at the suites - Day 50 - and the first day I can be home FOR GOOD. No plans of returns to the hospital or more treatments. A few tests and appointments here and there, but nothing I can't live with. In fact, right now I welcome the tests and checks because they all show signs of improvement and that's something I can definitely look forward to

Casey - *I am so happy you are doing so well and can't wait to spend some time laughing and having fun with you this summer!*
Gail - *Praise God. You Truly Are An Inspiration. Thanks for Allowing Us The Opportunity To Go Through This Very Difficult Journey With You. Love You, Gail*

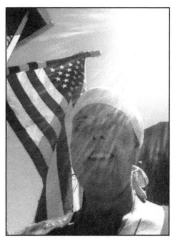

Mary - *I have learned so much from your journey Jenn. Not the least of which is to appreciate all the small things that I take for granted. We are so blessed to have the standard of living that we have, and I need to reflect on that and be grateful for it. It can be taken away in a heartbeat. God bless you and keep you strong as you complete this journey.*
Julie - *So happy for Jennifer. Cannot tell you how much I appreciate you sharing what you have been going through. God Bless and may the end of this healing journey be strong and uplifting for you.*

Cancer? What Cancer?
Jun 3, 2014

A week ago Friday I had my first bone marrow biopsy. That's where they collect bone marrow and stem cells from my hip to be tested for many things including any sign of the Leukemia. I've been anxious ever since wondering if this phase was truly over and if I was really going to return to normal life again. Honestly, I've been scared to death and haven't allowed myself to think about it much. I don't have any control over it anyway, but thinking the cancer had returned and I'd have to re-endure the past 6 months all over again was terrifying. However, the news was the best...No Sign of Cancer! My counts are all doing what they're supposed to be doing and I've been cleared to work in the fall. I still have a long road ahead with biopsies every 30 days for a while and my check-in appointments. But today I couldn't be happier!!

Rex - THANK GOD JENNIFER...I couldn't be any happier than I am right now knowing you are on the road to a full recovery from this insidious leukemia disease. Love ya lots, DAD ;-)
Jeana - I'm SO HAPPY for you Jen!!!!
Rosy - <3 <3 <3 Happy Dance! <3 <3 <3
Gail - God Is So Awesome and So Are You.

Good and bad hair days
Jun 14, 2014

The other day when my mom came to visit, she brought me a scrapbook with pictures she'd been taking since the beginning of this ordeal. It was amazing to look back and see the road I'd traveled, and I'm so glad she took the time to document it all. It'll be a timeless and precious treasure we can share, and as much as I may want to forget much of this experience, I need to remember what happened. And as I looked at the pictures, I realized that I was smiling in most of them, sometimes even a forced one, and in the others, I was clueless of anything going on around me. It made me start thinking about how truly difficult, horrific, appalling, destructive, and miserable it was. Not just on me, but my whole family who witnessed it. Absolutely heartbreaking for them as I endured the most heinous, inhumane, and inconceivable treatment one can imagine. I know I'm beating the odds, healing faster, fully recovering, feeling and looking great, and so on and so on. And I've been as positive as a person can be through all of the agony. But there were, and will be to come, some REALLY BAD times.

When counting days, I've been in the hospital, at treatments, or anywhere else but home more days than I've been at home this entire year. In 6 months I've spent more time with doctors and nurses than with my own family. That, in itself, is staggering.

And when people ask me how I'm feeling, my answer has been, "some days are better than others", like good and bad hair days. It was the same in the hospital, but most days were bad. And each day brought something different than the day before and was totally unpredictable. I had NO control over anything my body was doing or experiencing on the inside, but had to fight with the effects of it on the outside. The excruciating headaches lasted for days at a time, even when I slept, made my whole body hurt, and only softened with painkillers that made me "check out". It was horrible. My emotions were all over the place and my mood swings were vicious. I cried a lot, with reason and without. If I wasn't nauseated, I was running to the bathroom or commode, the most humiliating thing ever. After treatments, I just curled up in my bed and restlessly slept. There were rashes all over that made me itch so bad I was given sedatives so I'd go to sleep and stop itching. One of the painkillers gave me uncontrollable spasms and twitches, kind of like Tourette's, but with my arms and legs. That was torture. My fingertips were numb for 5 months and I still have some occasional, residual tingling. In addition to losing all of my hair, which thankfully now is growing back, I may lose my finger and toe nails. It hasn't happened yet, but like the rings on a tree marking years, my fingernails have depressions in them marking all four of my chemo and radiation therapies.

And the radiation. It almost killed me. It was necessary to have extremely high dose, full-body radiation, and the effects were monstrous. It was described to me like getting a severe sunburn, with blisters and all, from the inside out. It affects all the organs (liver, stomach, kidneys, lungs, intestines...) and is brutal on the mouth and throat. The reaction I had was "one of the worst" the doctors had ever seen. Good to know because it was the worst kind of agony I'd ever known. Because of the mucositis in my mouth and throat (swelling, blisters, and pain), which indicated how bad things were on the inside as well, I couldn't eat or drink, breathing was a challenge, I couldn't sleep, and I couldn't talk. I had to use a suction tool because swallowing was impossible. It got so bad the doctors almost put me on a respirator. Instead they put me on self-dosing Morphine, which was both great and terrible. As soon as I pushed the button I was out for hours and wasn't aware of the pain and trauma. And when I was up, I wasn't. My guests told me I'd fall asleep sitting up, in the middle of a sentence or conversation, during doctor visits and vitals, holding the suction tool...you name it, I slept through it or interrupted it. And I hallucinated not knowing where I was or who was with me. One night when John was visiting, he was so upset by it he had to leave because he didn't understand why, and couldn't handle mom passing out in the middle of the conversation. Horrifying to both of us - something I'd never want him to see, and something I'm sure he'd rather never seen. And this is just how I remember it. I'm sure my family can tell a far different, sad, and horrible story of what really happened. It's like childbirth; the pain you endure all goes away after the baby is there. My memories are fading as time passes and I heal.

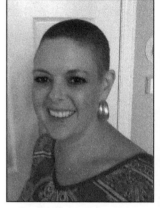

I'm past all that now, except in the pictures and as fading thoughts. As I recover, some days are bad hair days, but more and more have been good hair days. And in moving on, I still have fears that something will block my remarkable recovery. But I can't predict any of it and so I live one day at a time, enjoying my family and friends, and trying to live a purposeful and happy life.

Rex - Jennifer - This insightful review of your ordeal battling through leukemia is not only extremely accurate & heart felt but it reflects how painfully aware you were of every little detail going on in you, around you & for those who witnessed & endured the day to day battle in your courageous mission to survive! We love you dearly & are now more hopeful than ever of a complete RECOVERY & full REMISSION from this insidious disease they simply call ALL!
Gail - As I Have Said Before, Your Story Is So Touching and Means So Much to Me. You Have Allowed Us to Experience Your Difficult Times and The Good Times. I Hope None of Your Family or Friend Ever Have to Endure What You've Been Through but You Have Taught Us To Be More Caring And Compassionate For Anyone Going Through A Terrible Illness. Thank You Again for Sharing. Love Gail
Jill - I always knew you kicked ass. This is yet another example of how incredible you are.

Mary - *As I grow older, I realize that more and more of my friends and family have fought cancer. Thanks to your eloquent and heart wrenching posts, Jenn, I have an insight as to what that really means. You truly have had a battle on your hands, and although you have a magnificent and supportive family and circle of friends; at the end of the day it was your battle to fight. You have done so with humanity and dignity. Thank you for sharing your experience and I hope as these horrors you endured fade from memory, your appreciation for life shines on. God bless you Jennifer.*

Rene - *I can never imagine what you have been going through. You have the most marvelous way of expressing yourself. Thank you for sharing.*

Rex - *Jennifer your ATTITUDE & BEHAVIOR is an inspiration to us all! We are celebrating each & every day now because of what you have gone thru & your vision for the future...all "GOOD HAIR DAYS" on the horizon! Love you now & forever, DAD*

Soooo CLOSE!
Jul 16, 2014

I can't believe it's been since the middle of June that I last wrote a journal entry. It's been both fast and slow, easy and hard. A few weeks ago I had a major breakdown because I was just done with it all: medications and refills, the lack of clear communication with my doctors, the tedious and boring day-to-day monotony, I was tired of TV, books, games, and movies, and I couldn't do the things I would have normally done to break up or pass the time. I used to garden, camp, read, go to the pool and the movies, and many other activities that are just not reality for me right now. Too many dangers.

But once I got to Day 75, I started to see and talk about the end of phase two (recovery). Phase 1 was the transplant and all the treatments, phase 2 started when I came home for good, and phase 3 will start in 10 days. Yep, I'm on day 90 and looking back, can't believe it's only been 3 months since my transplant in April. That really made me see things in a different perspective. I am still early

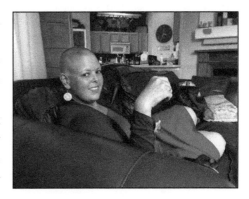

in the process, even though I'm feeling so good. But my getting back to as close to my previous normal will take more time, and I need to be patient with myself. I get so annoyed when I'm nauseous, or my hands shake (my handwriting has changed), or my mouth is constantly dry. Mostly side effects of the medications I take, but even that is coming to an end soon.

They say the first 100 days after transplant is like being a newborn - no hair, digestive problems, lack of immunities, what food I can/should eat, being weak and tired, and learning how to crawl again. Day 100 is like a birthday to toddlerhood and the thought process becomes what can a toddler do and eat? Where can they go? What are the safe boundaries? And I'm constantly asking myself those questions. It's so vague and defined at the same time it gets confusing.

I am scheduling daily outings with and without people and getting used to the stimuli all around me. Driving long and short distances, going to malls, lunches and dinners with friends, small parties and the like and it's been such a relief to have the contact with people. I am SO ready to be a toddler and explore the new reality I have been given. I'm not afraid of change because I know everything will work out. And I know I'll be able to handle anything thrown at me with patience and a deep breath. I was thrown into a fire and going through the fire it burnt off all the things and people and thoughts I don't need. I'm coming out clean and new on the other side, closer to my family, fully knowing who my friends are, and being comfortable with all of me. It feels pretty good.

Gail - I would love to go to lunch with you next week or even the week after. Let me know how your schedule looks. His. Gail
Janet - Way to go, Jennifer! I wish I lived closer so "we girls" (your mom too) could go out to lunch and have a giggle fest like old times. I am just so proud of you! You are really an inspiration, and something for the rest of us to think about when things aren't going like we want. I'll send some of Nolan's wedding pictures when I get them. Love and hugs, Janet

Latest Hurdle

Jul 21, 2014

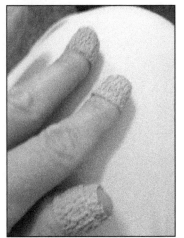

In the past 95 days I've recovered and healed very quickly and have been increasing my activities as I felt able. I've been doing housework (because living with 2 boys is a dirty job), running errands, meeting friends for chats, and working a little. And to be quite honest, I thought I was out of the woods with the debilitating, physical setbacks. I've been nauseous at times but I've learned to handle it so it's not really a problem. But this latest hurdle takes the cake.

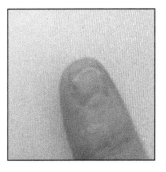

The chemo and radiation attack the soft cells first, hair, nails, mouth/throat, and organs. They told me I would lose my hair, which happened almost immediately, and that my nails might fall out. And it was kinda cool that I could feel tiny bumps in my nails, like the rings on a tree, for each chemo treatment I had. But now they are falling off, and I'm miserable. And I can no longer do all the things I had been doing because I can't get them wet, it hurts to put pressure on them, and they are falling off WAY below the cuticle. I'm having trouble texting on my phone because of the tape. Dressing myself is a struggle because my thumb nails keep bending back. Typing is painful, but I had to vent. I have to be ultra careful...again...because there's a real threat of "catching" an infection in the damaged and bleeding nails. The Dr.'s advice: tape, band aids, and nail polish to strengthen them. Are you kidding me? It might be God's way of telling me to slow down, take it easy. But I HATE this. I feel like it's thrown me back a month or so, and I'm mad. I've had 3 different types of tape and band aids today alone and can't find one that just doesn't fall off. If anyone has any suggestions, I'm all ears.

In spite of this, I can see how far I've come since I left the hospital. I'm going on walks, driving, eating, being social, and functioning in general. I can sleep all night, eat what I want, go where I want to go, and my flexibility (I can touch my toes again!) and endurance are improving. I have to remember I'm still an infant, at least for a few more days (5), and I can't expect to be all better only 3 months from the transplant. Patience, don't fail me now!!

Lopi - Have you tried gauze taped on? Clunky but padded? Let me know if you want me to come over and 'tape' you up. 😘

Kim - You can handle this, too. So you already know you can't do dishes, but make sure are not cooking as food is a huge source of bacteria. Plus, infants shouldn't cook and clean anyway. Prayers continue.

Rex - Only 5 days left honey to FREEDOM! I feel really bad about your fingernails hurting so much but just like some of the other horrible moments that this damn CANCER has put you through ... PERSEVERVE the best you can! This also will pass. God bless you, DAD

FREEDOM!!
Jul 25, 2014

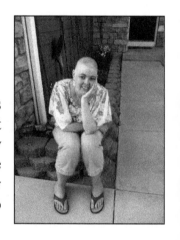

I made it to day 99, but what's a day or two? Day 100 is the magic number so tomorrow makes it official, but just like all those birthdays I thought I would feel differently (13, 16, 18, 21, 30...that's as far as I'll go), I'm pretty sure I won't feel much different. Just the next day in my new normal. However, it feels REALLY DAMN GOOD to have made it this far!!

It's the little things. I'm cancer free for 100 days! Next check isn't for another 3 months. I got my PICC line removed so no more cleaning the lines and no more syringes. No more showers with a shower sleeve protecting my PICC line from the

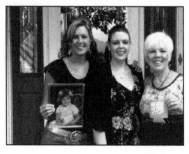

water. FREEDOM! They're weaning me off some of the meds with the worst side effects. I only have to see the Dr.'s 2 times a month alternating my Oncologist (Dr. Hyde who I LOVE) and Dr. Greggory who was responsible for the transplant. I can camp, fish, hike, work, travel, and do most things I've missed. I am so excited about the possibilities! I still have to be cautious, practice common sense, and wash my hands, but I have a whole new perspective on germs since this whole experience. There are things I wouldn't do and places I won't go for a million dollars.

And I can't wait for the 28th. I know it might seem early, but my mom, and sisters, Stephanie and Becky, and I are going to an Allison Kraus concert to celebrate. A girls' night out. It's in a relatively safe indoor venue and we LOVE Allison. Back to another tradition of normal we have done in the past. (A side note – Becky came down with a terrible cold and couldn't come with us, however we took her with us with this picture and in our hearts.)

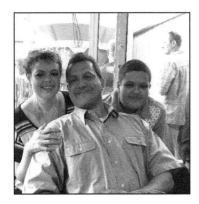

There are still some restrictions though. There are three things that can really set me back. It's the complications that can hurt me now. Molds and fungus are the worst thing for me because I could get a lung infection or pneumonia. So no gardening and stay away from dust. Sun is another thing I just can't risk. My meds make me sensitive to the sun in the first place, but getting a sunburn can trigger Host Vs. Graft Disease, which is an arch-enemy. It's like I had a regular transplant, like a kidney, and my body could reject the stem cells, attacking my liver, kidneys, and intestines. I can go out and do things in the sun but need to cover up and use sunscreen all the time. The third thing is infections or diseases. I've lost all immunities to everything I've been exposed to or had immunizations for since childhood. And I can't get them until the one-year mark in April. So I'll do the best I can to protect myself, but in the end, I really don't have much control over that at all.

All that being said, I wake up every day knowing today will be a mystery and different than the day before. I can schedule all the appointments and make all the plans I want, but life always has other plans. I listen to my body and do what I can, the best that I can. I test limits and boundaries because that's who I am and what I need to do to get stronger and healthier. But I also try to give myself the

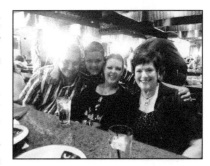

permission to be weaker, slower, and less able than I was, knowing it'll come back eventually.

I am excited to celebrate things like my son's birthday next week, to go out for meals, concerts, shopping. All with a bit less anxiety and much more happiness. My old reality is coming back a little at a time and I still have a lot of precautions I take (knowing how filthy the world is, taking hand sanitizer and wipes with me everywhere, choosing fresh), but it's worth the freedom I took for granted.

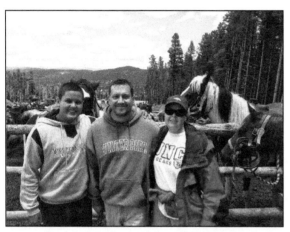

Next week I begin work again. Yes, it is soon, but I'm ready and will listen when my body speaks. I know my wonderful colleagues, friends, and co-workers at the district will support, understand, and show grace when I need it because they have since the beginning and I don't see it stopping now. Can you believe only 7 months ago I was given a morbid diagnosis, and today I'm thriving? It is still sinking in for me, a little at a time, and I have more and more flashbacks and memories of both the good and the bad days, But the good days outnumber the bad and I have nothing to really complain about. A new sense of freedom feels pretty good.

Rex - We're sooooo HAPPY HAPPY HAPPY 4 u Jenn!!!!! It's been a difficult 7 months but we hope that now u can get on w/ your NEW LIFE & PROSPER...Love always, DAD

Mary - I am so thrilled that you have arrived Jennifer! Those seven months will dim over time as the bounty of good days become your new normal. Congratulations on coming out on the other side where life is GOOD.

Rene - Congratulations! I am so happy for you and your family.

Valerie - As I stated in my previous message to you, my friend, you are my hero! I have thought of you and you're journey often, through my own journey! You are one strong woman! I am so happy for you! Thank you for sharing your thoughts and feelings here with us, it really was inspiring! Hugs!!

Chapter 6

Adventures, Pit Stops,

and Engine Checks

Reality Check
Aug 9, 2014

I did it! I went back to work July 30th and made it through the first three days with flying colors. I couldn't have done it without the thoughtful and caring "demands" from my supervisor to go home when she noticed I was waning later in the day. She

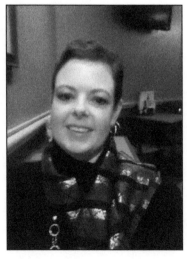 politely insisted I go home, take at least an hour break from all electronic devices, and knowing me, said I could work from home if I really wanted to, but no expectation to do so. I respect Karla so much and appreciate her understanding and knowledge and for taking care of me. Literally. She was always watching out for me and making sure I am ok. The job is secondary and my health and recovery come first. But she also respected my need to be normal and real again and include me in planning and training and decision making and leadership and all the other things I did before. I am exactly where I'm meant to be and doing exactly what I was meant to do.

This past week was a full week for me, and quite honestly, the best thing I could do. I was on the move and productive, using muscles and gaining endurance every day. Although they may seem like simple tasks, emailing and making copies, attending meetings and providing feedback, sitting at a desk, the up and down of filing and organizing, all take so much energy and concentration. The additional stimuli kinda hurts my brain sometimes and the chemo brain is NOT helping. I lose thoughts, and words so quickly. I can't multitask anymore or concentrate on more than one thing at a time. I often forget why I left my office, where my destination was, who I was talking about, or what I was doing. But I'm BACK! I'm taking things slow and easy, letting things go, putting off what can be done tomorrow, and not worrying about it - which is new for me. Things are not as important as they once seemed, and I'm so much happier, believe it or not. I find peace and contentment all the time. People ask me if I'm ok because I'm being quiet or pensive, but I am truly just being present and attentive and taking everything in. My intensity still exists and my attitude is always positive and geared toward problem solving, but I'm not driven to finish my list by the end of the day. It's easier than I ever thought possible to just let things go and know it will be ok. It's freeing on so many levels.

My reality is so close to normal again and I'm excited to be in the position I'm in. I've given myself permission to do what I can, the best that I can, and enjoy every day and every person in it. I. Am. Happy!

Joan - This is just awesome! I am so proud of you! Continued blessings as you start a new school year. I will be thinking of you. Hugs.

Rex - JENNIFER - I can't put into words (that are adequate) how we all feel about your miraculous recovery & being able to go back to work so soon in your continued recovery! I can hear & feel the excitement in your comments but also the peace, contentment & awareness of what you've been through & the acceptance of your current frail condition as you gain your strength back. Love you now & forever, DAD

Eldon - You are a real fighter. Even your toughest posts included a large dose of your positive attitude. Keep it up. A positive attitude will always serve you well. Best wishes.

Melissa - Yaaay

Steph - Jenn. You have always been my hero for what you can do. Now you get to be my hero for what you can let go, and the peace to be found there. You amaze me, sissy. I love you so much.....

Casey - You are so inspiring on so many levels! Keep that incredible attitude and thank your supervisors for proving people in a power of position can be truly caring for no other reason than being a good person. Love you lady!
Julie - Yay!
Kathy - It is so good to have you back! I pray for you each time I see you so make sure you wave your arms or something when you walk by me if I don't seem to have noticed you. Seeing you reminds me of God's Awesomeness!

Final Straw
Aug 12, 2014

Dear Leukemia,
Over the past 8 months I have endured many horrible things. Thanks to you, I have lost:
My hair
My fingernails
My flexibility and muscle tone
My endurance and stamina
My memory
My ideas and thoughts just float away never to be seen again
My taste and sometimes my appetite

But this is the final straw. BACON. You took away BACON?! It makes me sick every time I eat it. Doesn't matter what time of day or what I eat with it. Sick. I realized this about 4 weeks ago but refused to accept it. I thought maybe more time would make it better. But no. How can you do this to me? You've taken one of the major food groups away. EVERYTHING is better with BACON. You took away Jr. bacon cheeseburgers, and bacon and eggs (the phrase even starts with bacon. Having only eggs is just wrong), BLT's (again, STARTS with bacon), baked beans and bacon, turkey/bacon/avocado, and cobb salads, and that's just the tip of the iceberg. I'm heartbroken. I might just eat it anyway just to spite you...the taste is worth a little discomfort. Right?

Just like everything else you threw my way, I WILL overcome this too. But until then, this sucks!

Rex - *Maybe link or patty sausage will taste as good or better than bacon? Have you asked Becky if she likes bacon? Could be a stem cell transfer from your sister/donor! LOL*

Karen - *Everything is better with Bacon I agree maybe it's the nitrates in it that turns you off...hopefully this will ebb with time! Hang in there brave one!*

Steph - *This has gone TOO FAR. No one should lose bacon. Jenn, you can beat this. You can. You are strong. We are in this with you. Bacon doesn't know who it's messing with. We've got this, Jenn. One day we will sit around and laugh about how you had no hair and no bacon. They will both be back. I believe in you.*

Gail - *This is not funny but you sure make your miseries enjoyable to read. Love, Gail*

Rex - *OH OH...BAD NEWS JENN - I asked Becky if she liked BACON & she said she "prefers sausage" & that Marie doesn't like BACON @ all. LOL Your new stem cells might be telling you something huh? At least it's kinda funny! It's no wonder your hair grows (colic) in the opposite direction now. What's next...a yearning to get into real estate & become a property manager? HAHAHAHA*

Rene- *That is the pits! Perhaps turkey bacon even though we know that falls short of the real stuff.*

NORMAL-ISH
September

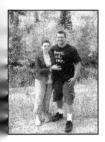 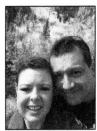

This month has been a whirlwind. I can't forget about the weekly blood checks and communications with my doctors, but they are quickly falling to the background and allowing life to come back, as much as it can. I'm going to John's football

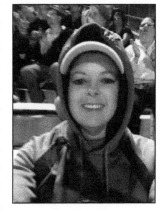

games. Joe and I celebrated our 15th anniversary with a quick trip to Silverthorne during the fall change of colors, which I couldn't help but reflect on the personal, physical, emotional, and relational changes (not to mention the hair!) I was experiencing. Although fall is typically known as a time of death, I see it as a normal change and preparation for change. I feel it exactly mirrors my experiences the past 6 months. First you are stripped of everything through chemo and radiation (the falling of the leaves, dying of plants - Fall), then there's a dormancy of the system as the body starts to heal from the inside out (Winter), and then the visual change of health and growth (new leaves, buds, flowers, color and green - Spring). That's where I am. I'm excited for the future and all the things I can do again and returning to a new state of the old normal.

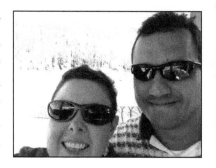

SIX MONTHS
Oct 19, 2014

I can't believe this marks 6 months! 6 months since my transplant. 6 months cancer free. 6 months in remission. 6 months. I'm so excited and doing so well it's remarkable. So many things have happened in 6 months it's hard to wrap my mind around it. 6 months ago it was Easter weekend and I had just spent the week enduring chemo and four high dose treatments of total-body radiation. I was scared to death...it shows in the pictures. I didn't know it then, but I see it clearly now. And I wasn't being *strong* or *fighting*, I was *surviving* the best I could each minute of each day. After the transplant, I thought I was going to die, literally not figuratively, and the doctors and my family weren't entirely convinced I would make it either. I was in so much pain, couldn't swallow, couldn't eat, couldn't talk, couldn't take the horse pills they were giving me and if things didn't improve I was going on a breathing machine, probably life support. Minute by minute I was watched, I couldn't function and morphine was my best friend. Thankfully I can only see it like a very foggy dream in snap shots, and more come to me each day. My family, on the other hand, saw things much differently. That week was agonizing for them as well. I was on the fence, could go either way, and didn't even know it. Scares the shit out of me now. There were 3 or 4 nights, since January 6th when I was diagnosed, that I was lucky to make it through the night, to include that first one. Their words, not mine. I didn't know it then, but the reality is sinking in really hard today. Enough of that for now...

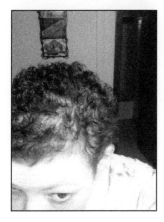Silly little things and slowly I'm getting back to a normal that I knew. Sometimes though, my little milestones bring with them new memories and emotions that sneak up on me without warning and I'm feeling things I didn't know were there. Like the 6 months deal that put me on the floor. So as I started driving to the salon to get a haircut and color today, I was almost giddy and had been looking forward to it all week. My hair is still rather short, but CURLY. Everyone was right, it did come back curly, and with more gray than I remember, probably thanks to Becky! And I didn't know what to do with it other than mousse, a flip with the fingers, and go. It didn't honestly matter to me what it looked like. I had Leukemia, right...who cares. But when I pulled into the lot and saw Tarah and walked to her booth, I lost it. It was SO familiar and good to be back, and it was one of the things I didn't know if I'd ever do it again. Seemed silly at the time, but I'm teary now just thinking about it again. The last hair cut I'd had was in the hospital room in January when they were shaving the rest of what was left of my hair off. Now you have it, now you don't. I cried then too, because it was a concrete "holy shit, this is really happening". And though I saw it as a blessing, my body's way of showing on the outside that the chemo was working on the inside, it was one of many firsts I never thought I'd experience in my lifetime. But I'm getting back to the firsts that make me happy, indicate my life is returning to an old comfort level, and marking each day as an adventure.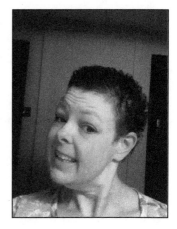

Walking into Mile High on opening day was magic and another first I was afraid I'd never see again. As I walked down the same tunnel I'd walked down for 20 years to my seats, I couldn't breathe. That stupid stadium had witnessed so much of my life and I felt like I was going home. It bounced me through my college drinking years when our neighbor fans probably wanted to throw us down the stairs. I think I spilled more than drank. It welcomed new family like Joe and John, watched others go. It's always been the way on opening day to hug and update the people next to us, all of us together, what had happened in the last year. Kids, and I mean KIDS, growing up, getting married, having kids, and starting businesses. Illnesses, not

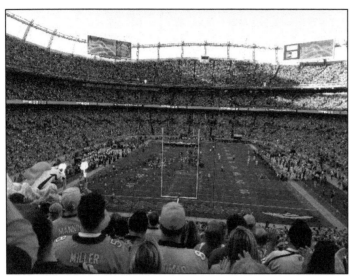

unlike mine, that we all endured for each other. And as I walked closer to the roar of the crowd, and slowly approached the end of the tunnel, and saw the stadium full of orange and loud and felt the energy of everything, yep, tear factory. And then the skydivers with nerves of steel started their journey into the stadium aiming for a window that must have seemed the size of a quarter, and I stood there for what seemed forever, just crying and smiling, and praying, and thankful, and happy. I took a LONG look at everything: the field, the fans, the scoreboards, the silly guys who dress up (even the creepy leprechaun dude and the orange pompom guys), Miles, the cheerleaders, the kickers practicing field goals, the sidelines...I took it all in like I had never done before. And it was a cacophony of what my heaven will look like. It was so beautiful (I'm crying again now thinking about it). When I missed the playoffs last winter, the thought really did enter my mind I'd never get back there. So being at the edge of the ramp and being fully immersed in my little piece of heaven was too much. And I felt my joy return, and for the first time, I felt like this could be my new reality too. But 6 months ago I wasn't sure I'd make it through the week. I've come so far and am constantly reminded what it was like a SHORT 6 months ago. I've been on the edge of every emotion possible, and sadness is quickly overtaken by joy and peace and tears of thanks.

I sent my sister (donor) a bouquet of orange roses today (well dad did it for me). It's because of her selflessness I am able to experience these new firsts, and I can't ever possibly thank her enough for her gift of life. We are 6 months old today, and I am like a child on Christmas Eve. So many firsts, some I can anticipate and most I won't. Like the curly hair! I'd like to say, "who knew?"...but I think we all knew Becky would make her mark somehow. And I'm thankful it's only the hair. I could wake up craving Diet Coke and Nicotine! LOL. And even that would be a blessing.

Rex - Jenn - That's the most beautiful commentary on survival that I have ever read in my entire life! Your visualization of your journey thru the life & near-death experiences of the leukemia treatments is unbelievable...especially your return to the Bronco stadium! I have no words to express my love for your contribution to all of us becoming a better & closer family as a result of your incredible battle for survival! Your legacy will live on forever honey? I love you SO much. What a journey. There are no words. I love you.

Angela - *Had to take a break from grading and now I am crying too hard to continue. You are an inspiration for all of us to look at life as a gift and cherish each moment like it may be your last. I am so happy for you and cannot wait to see your new Becky hair! We love you and think about you and no your family often.*

Gail - *Jen, we are so proud of you and happy to hear all of the wonderful new joys coming back into your world. Love to you and the family. Gail*

Amy - *Thank you for your heartfelt remembering. It's sometimes hard to look back but seeing how far you've come, it's awesome. God is always in the mix. I hope to meet you one of these days. I'll see if Steph can make it happen. Blessings to you as you continue to live life to its fullest.*

Mitch - *Jennifer you have been a "ROCK" in my life and your strength and courage are no surprise to me. You and your family have been in our prayers and we will continue to do so. God Bless You.*

Kathy - *Thank you for sharing your thoughts and experiences with us. Sometimes we ignore that we are blessed to even be able to get up and enter the day in a somewhat normal way. You have reminded me to count my blessings. God is blessing me by letting me have a chance to know you better. I'm glad we get to share a wall together!*

Giving Thanks
Nov 27, 2014

Thanksgiving. It's the same thing every year, isn't it? We wait for weeks, like a countdown, to get to the break from work. Which is exactly what it is. Then it's deciding whether to go somewhere or invite the world. Planning the meal (ham or turkey, pumpkin or pecan pie, mashed or sweet potatoes, casserole or fresh), shopping, stress, happiness, family, friends, hope. Then the day arrives and it begins with preparing a special breakfast, dishes, the parade, then more cooking. Throw in football, a beer or two, time with family or friends, and call it good. It's not even necessary to be present with people anymore with Facebook and Twitter, and smartphones to text a quick message or picture to loved ones saying "Happy Thanksgiving". Sit down to dinner and go around the table whipping off what we're thankful for that year: family, friends, a job, being an American, having the blessings of health or money or abilities or material possessions (personally I am thankful for warm showers EVERY DAY). Knowing things can be worse. At least that's what it's been for me, and probably many of us, until this year. A list of things to do; an obligatory moment to pause and bring to mind the things we are thankful for that we take for granted the other 364 days of the year.

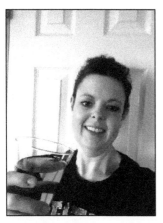

But not this year. I get it now. I am thankful. Period. The list is infinite and every day I can add something else. "Silly" things like turtlenecks or serious things like family. I've been thankful there was an available pump at the gas station, and thankful I can walk. Thankful for other peoples' grace and kindness, and thankful the dishes in the dishwasher were clean. Thankful for people in my life, and thankful people have left it. In reality it's all silly and simple. I am thankful. For every person I know, every conversation I have, every emotion I feel, every experience I have, every setback, every victory, every tear, every laugh, every moment of every day. As a human, I easily revert to reality and how the simple act of life overwhelms me shedding a cloud over what is really important. I worry. I plan. I speculate. I look ahead. But then I remember to breathe. That it will work out. That I don't have control and it's in someone else's hand. To stop worrying because what's the point? And some people think that's giving up or not fighting. I fight every day. I choose my battles. My dad always asks, "did I cause it, can I control it, can I change it?" With most things, the answer is no, I didn't cause it, can't change it, and can't control it, so I don't worry about it. When I am able to do that, I am filled with an instant sense of peace. It's hard to explain. But I prefer the contentment (NOT DEFEAT)

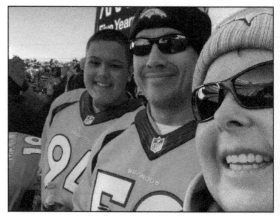

over fear or hopelessness or futility. I am a competitor and I hate to lose, but sometimes, giving up is simply making space and allowing other opportunities to tiptoe in and take hold. It gives me the moment to look at things from a new perspective and be thankful.

So today I am thankful. In every sense of the word, meaning, emotion, and intention. Peaceful, content, happy, hopeful, optimistic, gratified. Thankful.

Gail - Oh my. As always, I'm over overwhelmed with your wonderful way of telling your story. I'm glad it's late in the day as my makeup is a mess. Ha ha. You put it so beautifully. Life is so precious and so are you. Happy thanksgiving to all of you!
Melissa - So beautiful, Jenn.
Rex - Jenn - ME TOO ... You hit every nail right on the head honey. But mostly I'm thankful, grateful & humbled by your MIRACULOUS RECOVERY. Period. An INCREDIBLE JOURNEY ... I encourage you to publish your journal so that other people stricken w/ leukemia can better understand that there is indeed HOPE in the face of despair, pain & suffering. Jenn, you are the epitome of faith, hope & the power of prayer. You have given our whole family the courage to face life & death head-on & persevere whatever is thrown our way! IT'S A TOTAL "ACCEPTANCE" OF WHAT WE CANNOT CURE, CONTROL OR CHANGE. I feel I am well equipped now to live out my life in peace & serenity because you gave me the tools & confidence to know how to fulfill all of my hopes & dreams. You had the courage to look God right in the eye & let it be known that you were not ready to let go yet & he heard you loud & clear! He knows you have some unfinished business to do & it excites me to know your unfulfilled journey is still ahead of you! Get to work babe & do your thing. I plan to sit back & watch good things happen ... I've learned in my 70+ years to either lead, follow or get the hell out of the way! God Bless, DAD
Amy - Jennifer, Wow, you express what I think (sometimes, because I'm not always thinking about being thankful) so beautifully. You should consider writing a book. I love your humor, your humanness, your being open and raw and real. You remind me of the author, Anne Lamont. Thank you for letting me in your world. It has been an amazing journey but your blog is changing lives, too. On a side note, I have a dear friend that just found out their daughter, Kelly, who is 13, has Leukemia. She just left Children's Hospital yesterday. She set up a CaringBridge website, also. I would have never known about CaringBridge had I not known about you. Thank you.
Margaret - It was exactly one year ago that you came down to Houston to visit me and we laughed and laughed and had such a great time, yet several times you mentioned feeling weak. Then shortly thereafter, your world, and the world of the

countless people who love you, was turned upside down. Your strength, grit, tenacity and bravery throughout your battle with that horrible thing I will not dignify with a name, inspired and humbled so many, including me. I am grateful for you.

Valerie - I wish I could say "you took the words right out of my mouth", however that would be misleading because I cannot write like you! Everything that you expressed, I'm sure you know, is exactly the way I feel as well. Thank you for sharing! Happy holidays and God bless!

Anxiety
Dec 21, 2014

I am anxious. It's coming up on one year from my diagnosis January 6th, and I'm scared. The memories are flooding back, and with them the emotion that was disguised when it was actually happening. I see it like a movie, happening to someone else, and the feelings I should have been having at the time (fear, anger, pain) were covered by immediate and physical reactions instead. I wasn't worrying about the consequences or the risks because the complete shock of everything going on around me was overwhelming. The bells and the treatments, the doctors and the visitors, the chemo that took my mental awareness and logic, the medicines that created side-effects that then also had to be dealt with. I didn't process the fact that I had Leukemia. I didn't know what it was. Didn't have any sort of background experience to draw from. I was in the Dr.'s office, went to the emergency room, was told I had "it" but had NO idea what "it" was, and was admitted that night to have four blood transfusions just so I would make it through the night. Yep, I was that far gone.

But the emotions, the mental processing of information, the reality and the ramifications weren't gone; they were simmering under the surface and now they're presenting themselves every chance they can. Brief snapshots and flashes of my hospital room, sitting in the chair by the big bay window at dawn watching the sun light up the foothills, being pushed down the hall in a wheelchair to get an xray or procedure. Seeing myself in the mirror and not recognizing the reflection through the many stages of my transformation: hair, no hair, swollen, beaten up, scars and scabs and bruises. Remembering my mangled chest from an allergic reaction to the tape they had to use that created painful and ugly abrasions. Sleeping with my arm straight so my fluid lines wouldn't crimp and set off the buzzers. Being alone. Panic attacks when I couldn't get to sleep. Each visitor and the different things they brought me: company, holding my hand, food, watching a movie, prayer, safety, communion, comfort, pictures from home, clean laundry, laughter, good news, a pedicure, cards, optimism. Watching people taking naps in the chair by my bed and thankful for their presence. Being home but unable to do anything and spending hours of time on the couch watching tv and being bored. Re-learning how to walk up and down stairs. Watching one season slowly change into the next from my bed: winter, spring, summer. Catching up on "Orange is the New Black". Anticipating the infinitely long process of checking out and knowing I'd be coming back to check back in. Unpacking suitcases thoughtfully knowing I'd be repacking for the next trip. Nights that were more bizarre than others. Single events that took away my dignity or restored my faith. Being thankful I didn't have to wear a shower sleeve this morning or pee into a "hat" so they could compare my output with my input. Wishing I could (fill in the blank here ....).

And with each of those memories I experience a new emotion, most of them happy believe it or not. They bring a smile to my face and a happiness to my heart. Maybe it's because of the people, or the fact that I survived it and that's reason enough to smile. When I think about the times that were agonizing, the week they weren't sure I would make it through the radiation and thought about giving me a breathing tube, how my body was shutting down, the night my Hickman Line was pulled from my chest and the horror of watching my new stem cells flowing onto the bed and floor...all I can do is shake my head at the dreadful, eminent outcomes that didn't happen. And am thankful I can't imagine what my life would have been like if any of the decisions, tests, treatments, procedures, and medicines had a different outcome other than positive. Asking "what if" is as futile as asking "why". It doesn't matter I guess but I'm still scared.

Someone else's experiences and someone else's life. I guess when I really think about it, I'm scared in general of it happening again. I had no warning it was happening before so how do I know it's not happening again this very moment? I'm still processing words like Leukemia, remission, cancer, stem cell match, transplant, survivor, and future. It's like a bad joke. NO WAY did I have Leukemia. What is that? I really only said I "have" Leukemia for a few weeks, THANK GOD! I flew right through that stage and into remission stage. And the fact that I had an exact match. Are you kidding me? There are folks that have been in chemo for years waiting for a match and I get away with a 6 week wait?! And then transplant. And recovery, and back to work. Unbelievable. It's been less than year and as lucky, fortunate, blessed, thankful I am it was such a short amount of time, it also makes it harder to believe. It didn't have a chance to sink in. I didn't have to live with it long. It was like living with a bad haircut. A few weeks go by, the hair grows back, and you forget it even happened. People live in a world of "it can't happen to me", and so do I. Even now. I'm in denial so much of the time that when the memories come back, and the emotions hit full force, it knocks me down. It's a dangerous place to be because I take risks I shouldn't and have to remind myself to be more cautious. I forget I could get REALLY sick from a little thing and when that reality taps my shoulder, that's when the memories flash and I get scared again.

Now I'm on high alert for the things that they warned me could happen. I'm at a higher risk of getting a different cancer at any time, probably breast or mouth. My eyesight has changed and my 20/20 vision has become blurry. Cataracts are a real possibility. My teeth are sensitive and I could need a full mouth of dentures. Sounds sexy doesn't it? My mom teases that all that is perfectly normal to her. But she's almost 70 and that is normal for her. I'm 42 with a birthday next month and scared of becoming 70 at 43. I can't wait to be 70 when I'm 70, but not a day sooner. Maybe I'm afraid, not of these things in themselves, but the fact that every one of them reminds me that I in fact DID have cancer. It's real. And that is what I'm having a hard time processing. I don't know.

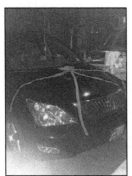 The fact of the matter is that in one short year, I had Leukemia, I became a cancer survivor, and I'm living a REALLY GOOD LIFE as real as I know how. I don't really believe in "someday" or "when" or "next time" any more and am living more in the today. I'm doing things as they come and experiences and people outweigh things (but I'm LOVING my new car!). The rest of the story is yet to be told. And I'll breathe through every memory and emotion as they come, especially this next month as one milestone after another pass by. At least this year I'll be home for my birthday and go to the playoffs and those darn Broncos owe me a Super Bowl!

Joan - Jen, you never cease to amaze me with your words, your spirit, the wonder of who you are. God gave me a gift when you came into my life so that I could better understand life. Blessings to you and yours this Christmas. (and I agree that the Broncos owe you)

Julie - Wow. Great post. Thanks for taking us on this journey with you.

Gail - Thanks again for sharing. We wish you and the family a very Blessed Christmas and a new year full of joy, happiness and new happy times with family and friends. Love you all. Gail and Jack

Melissa - Jenn, every time you write I am amazed at your ability to put your life into words. It's a gift and so are you!

Mary - I think what you are going through is a bit like mourning. That first year is a year of firsts. This is your first Christmas as a survivor, your first birthday as a survivor is coming up. No doubt, each of these experiences will be a time for reflection - and that's not a bad thing. You have been blessed with a year of firsts, and many more years after that. Thank you for sharing such a human and real experience Jennifer. You have enhanced my life through your words.Happy Christmas to you Jenn!

Jennifer - That makes a lot of sense Mary. You're a wise woman and I'm grateful for your thoughts. It's comforting to hear and makes me more accepting than anxious about the future.

Rene- Thanks for sharing all your thoughts and feelings. What a year! God is good. He must have something very special in mind for you.

New Year
Jan 6, 2015

One year ago today I went to the Dr. because I was feeling faint, couldn't breathe, and didn't feel well in general. After nearly leaving the office with a diagnosis and prescription for anxiety, my blood tests came back and were so alarming the Dr. sent me to the ER. Alarming? Hell, I was dying. Shouldn't have been walking, standing, driving. I was totally prepared for a blood transfusion to fix the "anemic" state I entered the hospital with. Maybe a night for observation and then back to life the next day. Worst case scenario, in my mind, was a blood clot or blockage that could be "fixed". But no, it was something far more sinister and evil and my life changed forever that day, and I don't know how to feel about it.

Is it a celebration? Hell yeah it is! I'm still here a year later. My life has resumed and I'm back to BC (before cancer) reality in SO many ways. I'm working full time. Driving. Sleeping. Going shopping and to restaurants. Being productive. Making meals and doing laundry. Being a mom and a wife. My list literally comes from what I COULDN'T do after the transplant. And as time passes I'll be able to do all the other things I missed last year and am looking forward to them like a new born or toddler would. First on my list is going to the Bronco Playoff game (Bowl Game?! haha!) this Sunday. And then my birthday. And then the Super Bowl IF things go my way. And then...

But it kinda doesn't make sense to celebrate the worst day of your life either. And it feels weird to be smiling when I think about some of the things that happened or came out of it. And it makes me cringe when I think about other times that were just down right agonizing. So today I'm going to be reflective and take the memories and emotions as they come and today will become tomorrow.

Now I'm living a new reality After Cancer (AC) that is somewhere in between BC, recovery, and AC. Yes, I'm working, but I also have to schedule in time for follow up appointments and blood draws. And appointments for the things that are now present as a result of the treatments. My vision is changing and thus am going to see the optometrist. Radiation knocked out my hormone system so I get to see the OB/GYN more frequently. My mouth still gets dry so there's gum everywhere. My immune system is still recovering and vulnerable and God bless me I don't catch whatever is going around, so I have hand sanitizer and sanitizing wipes everywhere too.

And when I think about these things, I just shake my head and shrug my shoulders because it's just the cards I have to play. The game changed from Texas Hold 'Em to War after the cards had been dealt, but I still have cards in my hand and will play them the best I can.

Gail - I truly hope someday you will publish your journal. It's is so inspiring. You are a role model for all of us. Love, Gail
Melissa - Jenn - Beautiful reflection on a special day by a beautiful person...you are the reason I want to live ... to share in your survival!
Rex - JENNIFER - We all went from counting the hours to counting the days then counting the months & now we can start counting the YEARS of survival, remission & a new beginning...one down & a lifetime to go honey! Love ya, your DADDY

What a difference a year can make!
Jan 19, 2015

One year ago today I was scared to death, sitting in the hospital, making the best of a birthday and praying I'd live to see another one. Prayer answered!!

THANK YOU! I couldn't be more thankful, more blessed, more happy if I tried. Reading your birthday notes fill my heart with joy and remind me how honored and lucky I am to know each of you. We may not have been in each other's' physical presence yesterday, but each comment gave me moments of time with each of you individually as I thought about you and treasured memories we shared together. You, my family and friends, should be celebrated for being the angels in my life. The cake picture is from last year, the others are from happier days since then....and I plan to have many, many more!!!

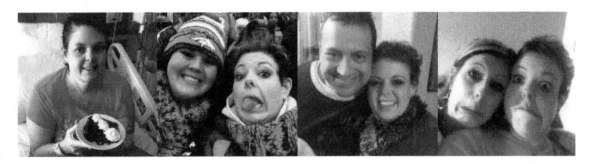

More fun times
Jan 19, 2015

Starting this time last year, people took pictures of my experiences while in the hospital documenting the good and the bad. Although I know there will still be bad, I'm focusing on the good and thought I'd post some pictures that represent my recovery and all the good I've experienced in the past year.

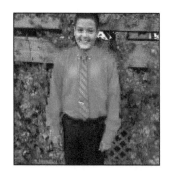 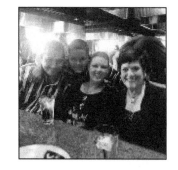 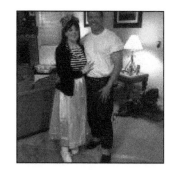

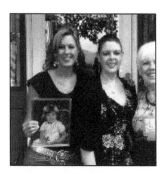 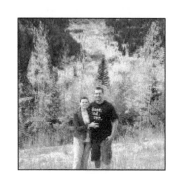 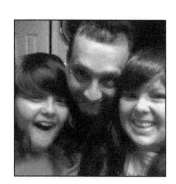

And more...
Jan 19, 2015

These make me so happy.

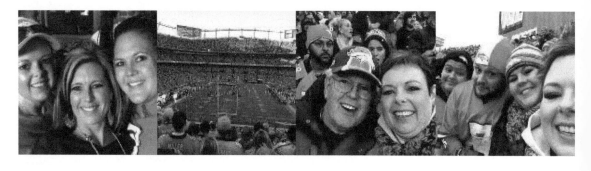

A year ago today...
Apr 16, 2015

I haven't written much this past 4 months because I thought you'd get tired of hearing the same old thing. "A year ago today I..." But truth be told, EVERY day the past 4 months has been a reminder of "A year ago today I...". I've measured every day since the January 6 diagnosis date by looking back at where I was or what stage of something I was in. I wrote in journals while in the hospital and as I read each day I realize all the craziness I lived through. The day to day survival. Just making sure the nurses were giving me the proper meds...of which I had to correct them many times - thank God for the lists in my journals. My moods, the various specialists, doctors, nurses, aides and visitors. Getting communion and praying with clergy. Weekly x-rays. Going to the bathroom maneuvering Phil (the pole with my hanging meds) and Flo (the machine that kept track of my vital signs) and all the tubes that connected us. Peeing into a plastic "hat" to measure my outtake. The amazing support from my family and the bickering, sharing, loving, giving, grace of everyone having a role. Mom made the schedule. Becky came on Thursdays. Ryan on Wednesdays and calling in the mornings (some of my favorite calls of all time. I still have them saved on voicemail). Mom and dad alternated the other days and Steph came in the evenings, during lunch, and randomly - sometimes with her kids in tow doing their homework in the lobby. Michelle who came when I needed a pedicure. Arranging the towels in the shower (three on the floor, two on the bench, one hanging) so I wouldn't slip, and wrapping my port with plastic and tape before every shower. Tedious. Putting on slippers every time I got out of the bed - you wouldn't want to fall down or slip you know. Sleeping with my arms in a certain position straight above my head so the squawking of the machine alarms wouldn't go off because of a blocked or kinked line. Remembering what baldness felt like...and kinda missing it. Being tired. Wanting to be alone. Wanting someone with me. Wanting to eat. Wanting anything but food. Sticking a suction tube in my mouth every few minutes to suction the mucus and saliva because I couldn't swallow anymore. Sitting on the death chair made of wood and a bicycle seat that looked like it came from mid-evil times for full body radiation. Felt like it too. All the seemingly silly celebrations but crying every time. Getting test results (positive or negative - however you want to look at it) that meant I was fighting the good fight. Trying to find something on TV to watch. Staring out the windows. I did that a lot. Praying. Watching the seasons turn as the tree buds turned into leaves. I sat in envy of that process while at the hospital in April wishing I could actually be outside and part of it. My participation in Lent this year was not a matter of giving up anything, I was rejoicing in all the things I had to give up last year and could enjoy this year. I was acknowledging my blessings every day.

All the milestones. First blood transfusion: January 7. First Chemo: January 11. Haircut to get rid of my remaining hair: January 23rd. February 1: first day home since going to the ER on January 6th. February 2nd: Broncos looked like idiots. February 5th: Repacking a bag for the hospital - this time I knew what I needed and what I wouldn't. I HAD to take my lamp. It made such a difference in making the sterile room feel homier. Everyone who walked in noticed the difference. February 6th: Checking back in for chemo part 2. Crying on the way there because I didn't want to go back. February 14th: packing Valentines bags for the nurses and delivering them with my magical cape a dear friend made for me flowing behind me. Even this snow today reminds me of a snow storm a year ago that killed my tulips and my flowering tree before I could see them.

March 27: The miracle of a perfect stem cell match with Becky. The next few weeks of tests and labs and appointments. Checking into the hospital April 11th to prepare for the transplant.

And April 16th. The last day of my old, diseased life. The last day. Ironically also on Christ's last day on earth - Holy Thursday. I was in a lot of pain from the radiation. My Mom and Dad were there the whole day, in and out, doing my laundry, taking naps, watching TV, observing all the checks I had to go through. Becky was suffering her own hell of pain from the meds they had to give her to stimulate her stem cell production. It was agony and thankfully Stephanie was there for her.

A year ago today...was my last day.

Rex - This is a BEAUTIFUL reflection & summary of your horrendous ordeal last year! Hope you can publish all of your journal entries, CaringBridge comments & the pictures of your battle with leukemia. It is inspiring & would be a great help to those going through the same miserable treatment & give them hope for their recovery. Your articulate view of the whole process is a gift from God & so are you Honey. Love ya now & forever, Dad

Eldon - A blessing from above. Best wishes

Steph - Happy birthday, Jenny!

Karen - You have definitely braved the storm of this hideous disease. Your journal needs to be in a book to help others it's truly inspiring and so are you!!

Rene - What a remarkable year you had and what amazing results. You have been blessed with such a wonderful caring family.

Gail - Love you and thank you so much for this beautiful recount of your amazing story.

Day 1
Apr 18, 2015

But today is my 1st birthday and I'm so stinking blessed. It's ONLY BEEN ONE YEAR since the transplant and I simply can't believe it. I was watching all of it through a movie lens so I'm sheltered by a foggy filter. But I know it was me. The pictures don't lie. The bald person staring back at me wasn't me. I want so badly to be the me from before, but I'm not, and I will never be. However, I can't believe how far I've come and am thankful every day for the little things. I can drive. My immunities are stronger (still fragile), but I'm so different than just 6-8 months ago. I can go out to dinner and order delivery and not be as afraid of the bacteria and other crawlies that would be a risk to my system. I can do movies, shop, and go to any public place. I've learned how to live differently, with hand sanitizer in every pocket, purse, bag, and room. I only eat freshly cooked food. I have fingernails again. I have eyebrows, eyelashes and hair again. I have more stamina and strength, but I am still weak and long days are hard for me. Showers without a cover are the schnizznit. Sleeping more than 4 hours at a time. I can walk. I have no pain. I can eat whatever I want - although my teeth and gums are now highly sensitive to cold and sweets so sugar is out. I can work in the yard again! All those things around the house that I used to look at and have to ignore because I couldn't do it and wouldn't ask for help.

I've decided to actually start doing all those things that I said "someday I will...". and being afraid of money suddenly didn't cause the problem it would have. And my priorities have changed. I care more about experiences with people. I bought a new to me Lexus for my birthday and Christmas. I deserve it. I participated in my

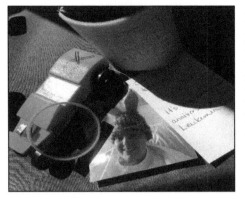

2nd Derby Car race, the first with happy memories of sanding the car with my dad when I was 10 and took 2nd! Beginners luck. It was my "Orange is the New Black" car representing Leukemia and that I'd beat it. I even wore matching sweats and shoes to complete the whole look. Look out next year, Uncle Jes! The 70th birthday/Easter party for my mom was epic and the entire family showed up;

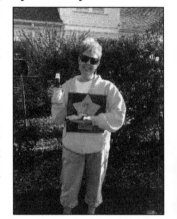

photographer and all. Everyone was there. All 22 of us. It was magical and beautiful and perfect.

I'm responding to invites I never would have - why not? We're spreading the love we felt during the time we needed it. I look at my work ID card and can't really recognize that person. That's both good and bad I guess. I still get so tired so fast. That's just annoying. But I can take naps at home.

I'm blessed and the reminders from Doctors that I am still an infant one year out of transplant really seems to bring home the truth. I'm still sick. I'm still fragile. I still have side effects and I am still recovering. Things will hold me back. But I'm way off the charts compared to their "normal" recovery and they really don't know what to do with me. So I get to do it my way. And this time, no one can tell me "that's not how we do it" or "we've never tried that before". Being that close to losing everything turns a potential risk into an opportunity again. Remember what it was like to be one year old? Curious about everything, not understanding no, climbing up on things because you could, making noise, demanding attention, questioning

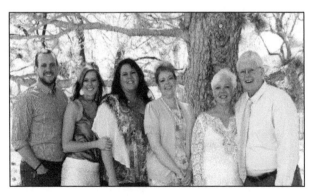

everything, awestruck by everything...thunder and lightning was exciting and new. Not caring what others felt about your clothes or your shoes or your words. In fact, everyone loved everything about you. Your mixed-up shoes and socks, the words that came out of your mouth without a filter, asking "why" about everything, still needing support when you fell, still needing help when you're tired, still needing help remembering the things that mattered, like food and a nap and cookies. Well, this 43-year-old - one year old still needs all those things. I might look like that beautiful Wedding cake on the outside, but inside they forgot the flower and sugar and I'm a mess.

But I'm only one and I have a lot to learn. :-)

Rex - Honey - You are NOT A MESS...in my world you are perfect & we all LOVE YOU just the way you are...being a one year old again is magical & a wonderful new experience! Try being 70 sometime & you'll appreciate getting another fresh start...enjoy your new beginning ok? Your loving father

Day 2: In the past year....
Apr 20, 2015

Today I started reading back to the very first journals I wrote. It put me in a very reflective, melancholy mood. I also cried a lot. And I feel there's a lot to add. I'm taking my time but I'll get through it. I want to add explanations, funny stories, reasoning behind decisions. Show pictures along the way and truly document my journey. Some other topics I want to cover are listed below and will get there in time. For now, I'm feeling enveloped by spirit and angels and in a safe place to allow those memories to surface. This women's retreat in Estes Park this weekend was no coincidence to me the very week of my transplant anniversary. And the topic is what season I'm in? A time to be born, a time to grow, a time to gather and a time to let go. I'm kinda all over the place, as I expected I would be. But I'm in exactly the right place. God carried me for a year. I had NOTHING. And he was there. My peace came from my faith it would all be ok. I woke up in the morning

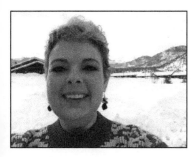 and sat in the chair by the window and looked at the Rocky Mountains, often covered with snow, and felt peaceful. I resented the door opening and interrupting my time with the mountains and in prayer or thought or just a conversation with God. I lived every day in those conversations. "Get me through this", with every needle prick, test, procedure and annoying Dr. visit. He's all I had and all I needed.

And when I got home from the hospital I knew how lucky I was to have had that time with myself, my family, and my faith. I felt terrific and didn't want to lose the peace and contentment I'd come accustomed to. There is something so freeing about being able to say, and BELIEVE, that it will all work out. It would be ok. Simply saying those words when I started to worry about anything made my life easy. I literally took a deep breath and had a physiological response to those words and instantly found my peace again. And when I went back to work and found myself worrying about work, or dinner, or John, I'd be able to say those words and I was ok. As time has passed though, I've had to say those words more and more before I felt the peace again. And at the retreat this weekend I discovered that I had moved further from my faith and my happiness. Somewhere along this journey I have forgotten who is the number one, and it's not me. It's like we broke up. I used to wake up and pray in the shower and spend my first moments with God, but lately I realized I haven't been doing that. I just started attacking my day and making plans and worrying. And other people's lives and drama have taken the place of that peace and I've fallen out of my joy.

Having had that epiphany, I made a conscious decision to stop trying to fix things, to stop taking ownership of other people's problems, and to keep things simple. And the moment I did that, I found my joy again. I found my peace. And I found God again. Life is easy again. I can shrug my shoulders again and say I don't know and not feel like I need to find the answer or fix it. I was starting to care too much about what other people thought about me, and I'm back to not caring, and I don't mean that in a negative way. Worry is a bad word and I don't want it in my life anymore.

So God and I talked and we've ironed things out and we're not broken up anymore. He comes first, which ironically puts me first. Crazy how that works.

So in future journals I want to talk about going back to work, all the travel I've been able to do, the wonderful events and celebrations and birthdays I've been able to go to, making experiences more important than things, my continued blessings, and how I decided that "someday" is now or never.

Gail - God truly is or only real strength. Hugs, Gail

Day 6 - It's the little things
Apr 22, 2015

The great and the not so great. My new normal showed back up. I've been taking care of tests and celebrating my one-year anniversary of being cancer free and was humming along just happy as a clam. REMISSION. CURED. And moving forward with things like immunizations. Well, I knew it couldn't be that easy, right? It's been about ten days now and I've been having a slight reaction to my one-year immunizations. I thought it was the Graft vs. Host being reactivated or something like that because I was having similar side effects like nausea and "stuff" and was managing it like usual. But Tuesday I woke up with half my face swollen to hideous

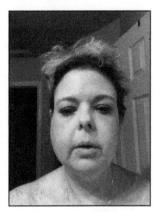

proportions and in incredible pain. I couldn't eat or chew, I was having stomach cramps, and was hating life in general. Luckily I had an appointment with Dr. Hyde that afternoon and he confirmed I had an infection in my parotid gland that was probably related to the shots and my system being vulnerable again. Those damn shots reduced my immunity instead of boosting it and now I'm a mess. And my sensitive system is purging the antibiotics with gusto - if you know what I mean. UGH! I couldn't go to work today and I'm on 2 weeks travel restrictions (I'll get back to that).

Of course my first thought was work. I almost started to panic but I was so proud of myself when I said "it'll be ok" and just did what I needed to do. I was scheduled to be in 6 teachers' classrooms today to administer the Advanced Placement Pre-Administration Session where they fill out the answer sheet with their personal and school information before the test to save time at the test. It is tedious and long and it takes time from the teachers and it's a just a necessary pain. Instead of freaking out about it though or worrying what the teachers would think, I emailed them and rescheduled it for Friday. There's nothing I can do so I'm not going to worry about it. I know this sounds little, but it was a big step for me. I don't have to be super Jenn. I'm pretty super just being Jenn!

Blessings in disguise: I was honored this year of being selected to be a trainer for the AVID program Summer Institutes this summer. I would be teaching other teachers the AVID teaching strategies and possibly going to fun places like Hawaii or Orlando or San Diego for the trainings. And it's a great gig money wise for 4 days of work. It's a really big deal in my work circles and I was really excited to attend the training to be a trainer this weekend in San Diego. Well...that's not going to happen after all because of the travel restrictions. At first I was really disappointed, but then I realized how much extra work and worry it had been putting on my plate the past 3 weeks. There was so much pre-work and hours of training videos, and a syllabus 33 pages long and..... I wasn't keeping up and actually started to panic a bit. But it's such a big relief! I have enough to plan for with my own district this summer and taking 54 people to our Denver training. That's plenty and realizing that, I was able to take another deep breath and be thankful for the little things. I'll try again next year, and chances are good that having been selected this year, I'll be "IN". And if I'm not, oh well. I don't need all that. Simple keeps me happy. And what do you know...NOT going to San Diego freed up Friday so I can do the AP stuff in classrooms without having to worry about finding a day next week that worked for all of us. Funny how those things just work out if you let them....

And now I have the treasure of time again. I'm hanging out in bed, reflecting on life, happy, and praying I make it to the bathroom in time. It's the little things, you know?

Kathy - Jenn, I am here and my work load is light right now. If there is anything that I can do to help out, please let me know. Until negotiations are over I can't do contracts so I am just doing things that have been put on the back burner for probably that last 20 years. If they could go that long, they will be fine to be placed on the back burner again. If you can't think of anything, I'll be here later (God willing). In the meantime, I will hold up the wall! I'm praying for you!

Rex - Jenn - I completely understand the little stuff... like getting to the bathroom in time (after shock of my prostate cancer), being able to tie my shoes (too fat), not having to put both feet on one stair tread at a time (2 torn meniscus), being able to hear people talk (new hearing aids), no more drippy nose & itchy eyes (Springtime allergies) ...life is good...sometimes but sometimes NOT. LOL Your gimpy rickety Father

Chapter 7

Hit and Run

Back to the ER
Apr 26, 2015

Dr. Hyde's diagnosis of an infection in my parotid gland in my jaw was right on and the antibiotics he gave me worked instantly. No more swollen cheek and my face looks fine again. But the antibiotics worsened my other symptoms and I'm headed to the ER. I've haven't been eating because it makes my stomach hurt and anything I eat or drink goes right through me. I started throwing up too on Friday. So after 2 nights in the bathroom and no sleep, and nothing substantial to eat but lots of liquids I'm losing all too fast, I'm headed in. Let's see what they say and if they can get this diarrhea to stop.

I did have two realizations this week.
#1. The shopping service offered by Walmart is LEGIT people! We needed a ton of things and I couldn't get to the store so I remembered the Walmart commercial that allowed you to order and pay online and deliver to your schedule. As ridiculous as it sounds, I tried it and it was awesome. We got our milk and eggs and yogurt and Cascade the next day delivered by the nicest man and even got 2 big boxes of trial size gifts. It's not something I plan on using regularly, but Walmart Grocery has a new fan.

#2. I might think I'm done with Leukemia, but Leukemia isn't done with me yet. I'm still only a year old with year-old liver, kidneys, skin, digestion, etc., and everything else like vision and memory and hormones are like that of a 60-year-old.

My body doesn't know what to do with itself and I'm doing pretty damn amazing considering. I'd like to just move on and forget this ever happened, but it's making every effort it can to stick around and remind me. Although I've been doing laundry and dishes and working in the yard, I really shouldn't be. I could've gotten a bacterial or viral infection from any one of those things, and it could be worse. And I guess I still need to ask for help.

It's also making me realize that this summer and all my "next year when I'm healthy" plans are not going to be back to old normal. I feel like I missed so many things I want to get them all in this summer. But I need to take things slower and that frustrates me. I have a half-demolished deck in the back I wanted to make into a vegetable garden but it's not looking good - literally and figuratively. I wanted to go camping, a lot, and am not sure that, the boating, or the dirt biking are going to happen either. I'm looking forward to finishing a full year of school/work and will be done in 5 weeks...a tremendous accomplishment not to be overlooked or down played. But once again I'm feeling restricted and imprisoned and I don't like it one bit. So off to the ER to get some magic fluids and hopefully some answers.

One last thing, but probably the most important: thank you to all the people who stopped in "just because" yesterday. As much as I didn't want to plan anything and just sit on the couch waiting for the next bathroom sprint, seeing my sister Becky and my nieces, and having a good friend bring me some protein powder and much needed hugs, made my day, and makes me smile now. I value those reminders of the good things that Leukemia gave me even more than the bad. They make the bad seem not so bad.

Rex - Jennifer - We're glad you decided to go back to the ER @ the hospital honey. At least you'll get re-hydrated & some tests to better understand what's going inside your delicate bod! Those recent immunization shots may have had something to do with this goofy reaction going on? In the meantime...till we find out the results of your tests...get well & get back on your track to a full recovery to your "NEW NORMAL" ok? Love ya, Mom & Dad
Kari - Praying for you!!! Please let me know if you need anything!! Love and hugs to you!!
Margaret - Damn it! But knowing you, it's always "one step back, TWO steps forward." This will pass! Love to you, Joe and my favorite boy on the planet. John.
Julie - wondering how it went and how you are today. Thinking of ya

Home
Apr 26, 2015

Well they took blood and other samples and didn't find anything abnormal. No sign of bacterial or viral anything. No new meds. Blood counts are ok. Sending us home with a pat on the back. I'm so relieved it's "nothing" to worry about, but now what? I'm still going to worry and wish I had something concrete to treat. As it is I'll be taking Imodium, eating what I can, drinking lots of fluids and trying to keep my probiotics safe and balanced.

Thank you to everyone for helping out during this weird week. I guess we'll just see how today goes.

Graft vs. Host Disease
Jun 2, 2015

So all the tests and doctors have confirmed it; I have Graft vs. Host Disease and they are insanely happy about it. I, on the other hand, am miserable and have been for weeks. Maybe even months. They say it's good to have GVH because it proves my new stem cells and immune system are running beautifully. I'm sorry, but I'm just not seeing it...literally. The GVH presents itself by attacking my soft tissues: eyes, skin, mouth, and organs. So I have a hives-like skin rash, small blisters in my mouth, and eye issues. My eyes are so irritated the whites are swollen and red and painful and they sting all the time. I can't focus on much at all. I go through a bottle of Thera Tears every week. I'm wearing sunglasses inside and out. I look like a damn cartoon character. The best way to explain it is squinting through a day with soap in your eyes. It wears on every cell and process in my body. I'm not only body exhausted, but brain exhausted too. I'm extremely depressed and feeling like I'm back to last summer with lots of things I want to do, and have time to do, but can't do. The pool - going shopping for a suit that fits sounds like torture. And sun will make the GVH mad and set off another reaction. I've got my fishing poles all ready to go, but again, going to get a fishing license sounds like hell on earth. There are so many fun little yard projects to do...but...

Wouldn't it be nice to have a "wish list" that actually got done through wishes? I would love for the tree ring in front to magically appear. Or the veggie garden replacing a worn-out deck to just be done. Flowers should just plant themselves - where is that garden fairy? Hello???? Ok, back to reality.

I feel like my whole life is spiraling out of control. Everything is off balance in a bad way and I'm very lost. I'm supposed to move my office out of the administration building and back to the high school, but they don't have a place for me. So my office is packed in the back of my car with nowhere to go. I know it's summer so I guess I should be happy, but I do not like being homeless and uncertain and unwanted. Last summer at least I knew where my home was going to be when I got back.

I hate my new normal. And I probably shouldn't be writing this or making it public. Unfortunately I know there are people that will use it against me instead of seeing it as me letting my guard down and being honest but I really kinda don't care. I hate feeling, seeming, looking, or acting weak, but that's all I feel I have right now. I hate questioning myself, my actions, and my decisions. I'm not sure which is worse; having mental and physical capabilities and not being able to use them, or not have the capabilities and wishing I did but couldn't use them if I did. I'm crazy for admitting it I know, but there are days when I kinda wish I was back in the hospital. Things were actually simpler. And as much as I hated being there, I really enjoyed the time with family, and contentedly staring out the window, and not having much to worry about. It didn't matter if I couldn't see or think straight. It wasn't important if I achieved or accomplished anything more than getting more than 2-3 hours of sleep. Thank God cause that Chemo Brain thing is very real.

Things could be worse, right? And they could be. And I am constantly counting my blessings and giving thanks for my family and friends and positive circumstances. The list is infinite. But forgive me for making fun, I'm seriously just not seeing much good past the nose on my face these days. Hopefully tomorrow things will be more clear.

Rex - *Honey - I'm glad that you're finally opening to the reality of your recovery & VENTING in such a heart-felt manner! This a very healthy & genuine way to expose your feelings & grief to all of us .... Please don't ever regret expressing how you really feel ok? I love that you are so able & willing to expose your life as it really is ... battling this Graft vs Host Disease is just another chapter in your survival book that you are dealing with in a very understanding yet I know a very painful way! Forget about the wish list & concentrate on whining & battling thru this ok? Just try to gut it out & know that we all love to you & know that Dr. Hyde & others are always there for you no matter what! Most of all...I am living this episode of genuine HATE for what you're going thru right with you like it or not! Love ya now & forever, Dad p.s. I HATE CANCER & I HATE WHAT YOU ARE GOING THROUGH RIGHT NOW! GRRRRR*

Kari - Praying for you Jenn and sending hugs!!!! I'm so sorry you have to go through this-it's total BS! Please let me know if I can do anything to help!!!! Xoxoxo!

Tammy - I have no idea what you must be going through, but know that I think of you frequently and I say a prayer for healing every time. I hope tomorrow is better.

Kim - I am so sorry you are having to deal with yet another complication of this process. I am glad that at least the doctors are happy. Please know that I am sending my prayers.

Katie - Your 2nd to last paragraph breaks my heart. You are a strong lady -keep shouting it from the mountain tops!

Gail - Wow. What a mess. You are in our prayers and I can't imagine how you feel. Will the Graft disease get better or is this for a long time? You are still my hero and even heroes deserve a pity party. Thanks as always for sharing your life and feelings with us. You are an amazing lady and I pray your life would level out soon. Love Gail

Janet - Oh Jenn! I'm so sorry! I'm thinking about the wonderful evening we all had together in Dallas so recently. You were feeling so good, and were so enthusiastic about your job. I am very teary reading about what is happening. I just hate this, as we all do! Hang in there! Lots of love, Janet

It's the Little Big Things
Jun 5, 2015

I don't think anyone would understand how amazing yesterday and today are to me. Although my physical setbacks make things much harder, it didn't matter one bit. You see, yesterday was Joe's birthday, but a year ago I was still recovering at the residence home and couldn't be here for him. I was fortunate that Keeley and Casey made him a beautiful home-cooked truck cake and was able to fill the void of my absence, but that was a HARD day! But not this year. I'm home. And Joe

128

took the week off and we've been spending some MUCH needed quality time to rediscover who we are. Figure out what our new normal looked like for us as a couple. Reconnect. And we went to the hills to have a prime rib and crab leg dinner, and wander the casinos, and dodge quarter size hail stones, and laugh and play and be silly and enjoy each other again. We clapped and high fived when we won a big one...you know, one of those penny machines that says you won 2000 credits which equals a whopping $20 bucks but keeps you playing. And celebrating each time we got a bonus or free spins. And Joe likes the Craps table. I found a VERY fun Willy Wonka machine that let me borrow about $100 - I say borrow because I won it and gave it back. Hey, at least we played all night, paid for the room, dinner, and had money in our pockets when we left. It was the best time ever. And nothing else mattered but him and me all day. I. WAS. HERE. On so many levels, I was here.

No one told me it would be like this....
Jun 14, 2015

I'm not going to lie. The past few months have been hard. Trying to pretend that things are normal is getting harder and harder. People keep asking me if I'm sick because my eyes are so red I look really sick even though I feel fairly good physically. I've been finding myself asking for "help" A LOT lately. It would be one thing if this Leukemia thing was really over and done when I got the Remission announcement, but it doesn't stop. Yesterday I had to pull over while driving because I honestly couldn't see anymore. My eyes stung so bad I couldn't open them and Joe had to take over...thankfully he was there to do so. Within a few minutes and eye drops later, I was on the mend, but exhausted. This is a daily thing and if the doctors didn't give me a little bit of hope that it would eventually go away altogether, I would be feeling rather hopeless. I can't really read what I'm writing so forgive the errors. Even that's a struggle these days. When's it going to end? I went fishing today and as much as it was a victory to be out, I couldn't tell if my rod was moving or not because I COULDN'T SEE it. And the joy goes out of everything quickly when frustration sets in.

Another realization I've had is that I and we still need help. Last year I was receiving notes and cards, and meals, and random gifts, and lots of thoughts and prayers because it was still all so new, and EACH gift of love was treasured beyond words. And it wasn't until just this past 2 weeks when I started getting little acts of kindness that I realized I still need those things. And Some good friends gave me a ride and treated me to a soccer game when I needed it. And Joe's co-workers gave him rides while his truck was in the shop. Out of the blue I received a card and note that couldn't have come on a better day. It was a huge lift and left me filled with hope and comfort again. I need help taking care of Sydney a few days this summer because she doesn't do well in kennels and we can't take her with us. I thought it was going to be impossible, but another angel volunteered to love on Sydney for us. Although the shock and the initial ordeal from last year is very much over, the recovery and aftermath are still very real and life imposing. And I can't believe how many times a day I say "I wish I knew someone who...", or "I wonder if anyone could help me...". Texts from people checking in are so appreciated. I feel really confused and lost and alone and there are days when I wish someone would just tell me what to eat, or where to go, or what to do. I'm putting up a good front and things probably look good on the outside, but I'm still scared all the time and never know what the day is going to hand me. The best laid plans are almost always interrupted, in the spirit of grace and acceptance, but it is still maddening to have goals that just aren't realized, and not for lack of planning or trying.

So thank you to all of you who are still sending your thoughts and prayers and making our lives easier in one way or another. I wouldn't be where I am today without you, and I'm finding I can't curl back into my comfortable world of independence and get through this alone either. I need the constant reminder of my frailty and your unforeseen kindness continues to overwhelm and comfort my worries, fears, and insecurities. I am forever grateful.

Rex - Uncertainty & fear of the unknown are the most difficult issues for most of us to deal with...I think we like to know what's going to happen so we can be in CONTROL of our own destiny. Unfortunately, life doesn't seem to lay it out like that so thank God for the gift of his grace through prayer. It's one reason I say to myself the "SERENITY PRAYER" & constantly work on my 'ACCEPTANCE" of the things & stuff I cannot control or have an effect on. This recovery period for you right now must hell but I know it will pass...in the meantime just "fake it till you make it" (an AA slogan) & know that we are all praying every moment of every day for God to grant you some peace & comfort...both mentally & physically. Love ya now & forever honey, Dad
Kari - Praying for you every day and will continue to do so! So sorry this is happening! Xoxo!

Joan - Jen, I wish I was there to hug you. How sad when we all get wrapped up in our lives, and the days go by, and we don't stop to think of others who might just need a simple smile. You are still such a warrior and I won't be so neglectful. Love you and prayers.

Karen - Dear Jen, just read your latest post. Throughout this journey you've been a warrior. I admire your strength, faith and the honest way you share your feelings. As difficult as this is you know how to do it ....one day at a time. Still sending prayers for you and the entire family from your Illinois family.

Another one
Jun 16, 2015

So yesterday was definitely in the top 10 of worst days ever. There just aren't the words to describe the absolute agony, helplessness, and hopelessness that I feel on those days. My eyes were so bad I couldn't open them. Tremendous pain. Stinging pain. Lots of "cant's"...can't drive, watch tv, leave the house, play games...

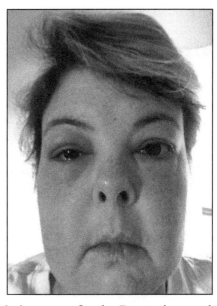

The only way I can explain it is trying to see with soap in your eyes or how it feels when pool chlorine wipes out all semblance of anything good and makes everything blurry and painful. And that doesn't even scratch the surface of reality.

And nothing so far helps. Antibiotic drops, steroid drops, refresh, Restasis, cool water rinses, ice, sleep, gels. And nothing I can avoid helps either... I've been walking around with no makeup, lotion, sun screen or anything else that could provoke a reaction... In my eyes that is. I'm getting plenty of reactions from people. Are u ok? I must look stoned or sick or whatever. And I'm tired of trying to explain it. I feel ugly as hell. Meth addicts look good compared to this.

And my poor John was so amazing. He gave me ice, hugs - like those soul filling hugs I gave him as a child when he was sick - made me food, pet my head, food and

131

water, reminded me to breathe. And all I could think of was how lucky I am to have him and curse the devil for making him experience this. And I lie in bed crying with no tears and desperation and prayers that this will go away. I even emailed my specialist only to get her auto-reply that she was in Hawaii and would be answering messages in July. Great. All alone with no answers.

I feel like I'm losing so much life again. All the things I was so excited to do are off the menu. My fishing poles and golf clubs are in the back of my car screaming to be used. All I can do is shout a soulful, gut wrenching, wail of sorrow that this will ever get better.

How am I supposed to live in the world of the healthy when I'm anything but? Drink because who cares? Eat cause I'm bored? Take a sleeping pill so I can sleep through it? I. Am. So. Lost.

If you see me, just know it's a strong front. Fake it till you make it, right? I'm just so pissed. I have a life to live. Things to do. Places to be. Experiences to have.

And I can't breathe. And I slowly feel goodness slipping away. So I'll grab it anywhere I can. The U.S. Women's soccer team plays tonight. Let's see if they can pull off a win and slip back into my happy zone.

Joan - *I wish I could do something, Jen. I will continue to pray and pray for you. What is causing all this eye pain?*
Rex - *BREATHE...PRAY...ACCEPT...HAVE FAITH...READ SCRIPTURE.. .EAT... DRINK...SWEAR...SCREAM... Whatever it takes to take to your mind off the pain honey. We're all feeling your suffering & helplessness...don't know what to do or say? GOD BLESS, Dad*
Derek - *Dear Jennifer, this is Derek writing (piggy backing on my mom's account because I can't keep track of a password to save my life). I'm so very sad and sorry to hear where you are right now, deep in a tunnel (again). I can't even imagine the frustration you must feel to be dragged back down to a point where the basic joys and activities of life are denied to you. If it is helpful at all to know that there is one more person in this world pissed off on your behalf, know that I'm that person. And I also have faith. Not necessarily the religious kind - sadly, I'm not a religious person - but rather faith in you and your family, the strongest, most resilient people I know. Your undeniable strength, your sense of humor, and yes, your faith in God*

will carry you through. I just hope you get through whatever this is as fast as hell.
Your friend, Derek

Summertime Blues and the Rainbow
Aug 16, 2015

I realize my last entry was a bit dark. And I haven't updated this for months because quite honestly, it got darker and life became a marathon of just surviving each and every day. Right after my last entry, things got serious. I began a barrage of doctor visits to various specialists to try to determine what was going on with my eyes. The whites were swollen and red, my vision was blurry at best, they hurt all the time, and I was literally disabled from doing most things other than stay in bed with ice on my eyes. Not the best way to spend a summer.

I started seeing an ophthalmologist to figure out why my eyes were so swollen. His diagnosis was heartbreaking and yet another blow from files of "things I caused". I've always had an allergy to our cat Serena, but we lived with it and it never seemed to really bother me before unless I pet her and stuck my fingers in my eyes. But now that my immune system was on hyper drive, the allergy was the prime culprit and I was "ordered" to find her a new home with the warning that the Dr. had seen people die rather than let their animals go. I was also given eye drop steroids and other

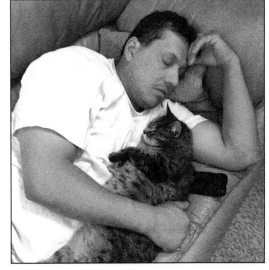

treatments I later stopped because they were just making things worse. But back to the cat...

She was Joe's baby. We had always thought I was the cat person and Joe was the dog person but we were so wrong. When we went to adopt Serena 15 years ago, I insisted Joe go with me to "approve" (help choose) our next pet. When we got to the adoption fair, it took all of 15 seconds for Serena to choose him. She looked right at him, started rubbing against his legs, made him pick her up, purring.... she put on the whole show. Done and done. I think she knew I had to keep a distance, so she made Joe all hers. She had him tied around every little paw and trained him to love her perfectly. When he came in the room or home from work, she'd start talking (yes, she talked) and would flop in the middle of the floor, belly up, inviting him to pet her. He was always more than willing to accommodate her and laid down right next to her on the floor. She'd follow him everywhere. When he sat on the couch, she was in his lap. When he slept she was in his arms. They were buddies.

So when I came home with the unbelievable news we were going to have to find her a new home, we were all devastated, and Joe was understandably in heart-gripping grief. And it was yet another agony I felt I caused my family. I didn't know how much more we could take. Joe got up Saturday morning and took her to the shelter with the belief they would have to put her down because of her age. I couldn't even look at him or her. I was broken that I had caused more hurt, again, and had no control over anything, physically or in my environment. It was a sad, sad time.

The good news? One of our neighbors down the street, who also adopted our hamster Chica when we couldn't keep her, took Serena home! She was one of the family the first night and has them all trained now too. And John can go see her whenever he wants. The one thing this past 2 years has taught me is to always look for the rainbow!

But the summer isn't over yet. Even though Serena's story has a happy ending, the series of events to follow were just as unbelievable and life changing. More later...

Rex - Jennifer - Like I've learned over many, many years of living with my own demons...if we can "LET GO & LET GOD" very often (with the help of prayers) we find the we're really NOT in charge here! What a relief honey...it's TRUE. Love ya always & forever, Dad
Kathy - Hang in there just as you've been doing for such a long time now. Happy news that Serena has a new home and it's just down the street. So sorry to hear the recent months have been so tough. The mid-west Walker-Dyers, Walker-Kehls et. al. have you covered with prayers. Take care.
Gail - Praying for the family. I think God knew you needed a good solution to Serena and Joe. Its hard many times but he is there looking over us. Love, Gail and Jack

More Rainbow
Aug 28, 2015

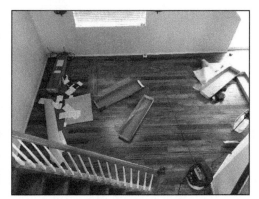

Well, moving the cat out to a new home to eliminate the allergy and hopefully relieve my GVHD symptoms of dry and swollen eyes and rashes, wasn't the end of the story. To play it safe and remove all the animal dander and hair and whatever was making me sick, we had to do a complete house remodel. That meant new carpet, floors, thorough vent cleaning, and deep cleaning for the house. What? Although our carpet was shot and needed replacement and the hardwoods needed to be sanded and refinished, and we had already discussed how much it needed to be done, we weren't ready for such a massive overhaul. We thought maybe one floor at a time? Maybe carpeting first? But we knew the impossible amount of hard work that would take and we just didn't have it in us. It would mean moving out until the work got done, a few weeks at least,

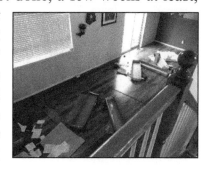

and who does that? Moves out of their house for repairs when your wife is very sick and you don't have the funds mostly due to the new medical bills? And we didn't have a place to start. WELL, this was one of the hardest bricks to the head I've ever received from God when he literally took control and made the impossible, possible. And largely due to Ryan's (my brother the insurance agent) contacts and Angel team!

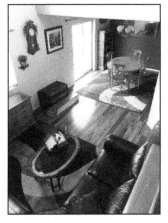

When you have to do this kind of full house cleanse, it's like you're moving out. We spent a week packing books, small furniture, closets, emptying shelves; just like we were moving. Then Ryan's team went to work. His team is comprised of other small business owners who use each other as references, but also believe in giving back to the community. When Ryan told them my story, they dropped everything, even during this busy time of their "season", to get this done ASAP. The first team moved all the furniture out and into the garage. Two days later a new crew removed the carpet and floors, next team installed the carpet and new flooring. The cleaners not only came after 5:00 on a Friday, they left me 2 beautiful flower arrangements. Bring in the vent cleaners (a full 10-hour day doing a thorough scrub). And lastly the movers to bring back in all the furniture. They were our angel team and couldn't have done it without them, OR my parents who took over the operation, contacted and communicated with the companies, scheduled the teams AND drove up from Colorado Springs to let the teams in and out! I made this sound all very easy, but it was 4 weeks of hell. Plain and simple. Yet another "thing I caused". More agony for me and my family and I couldn't do a thing about it.

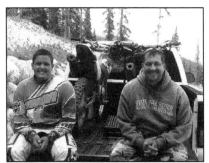

And God really knows when to pull the trigger when the time comes. We had been set up with Domis Pachis, a NFP group in Summit County (Breckenridge area) that donates meals, time, and housing for respites for cancer patients and their caregivers. What a blessing, in all ways. Joe, John, and I were able to enjoy the 1.5 million dollar "vacation house" for a full week while enjoying pre-made meals, using donated coupons and gift certificates for meals and fun stuff, and all while the house in Thornton was being demolished. We loved our time in this astoundingly beautiful home, but it wasn't our home and our home was being pulled apart. Bitter-sweet, but the best scenario ever to get me safely out of the house! When we got home they were still installing the floors and carpet. Joe wanted to stay, but I couldn't so I had to find an alternate place to stay. And... tadaaa... there the Gallagher's' were again saving the day. They were leaving on their 2-week road trip and said I could stay at their place as long as I needed to. Again feeling unbelievably blessed, I was there for nearly 2 weeks. At that point it was time for

my AVID conference in downtown Denver and got to enjoy a special treat of staying at Ryan's for a week while the house aired to safe levels and I could be close to my work responsibilities. Yep, four weeks living out of a suitcase. During the months I'm supposed to be getting rest and recovering from a hard 18 months. Terrific timing of events, icky reasons, and best possible outcomes.

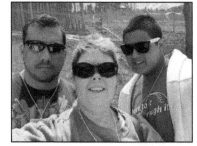

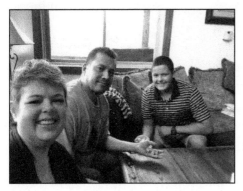

So when I returned home, I couldn't believe it was mine! It looked beautiful. I was in a new home and hoping for a new start. We went shopping for new furniture - yes that had to be thrown out too - and floor rugs and redecorated and it's beautiful. Far from being paid for, but beautiful and home. Once again we went through the unbelievably hard and came out feeling blessed and thankful.

Kim – You are an incredibly brave woman. Prayers said. Hoping that things smooth out for you now.

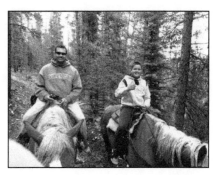

It's the rain that makes the rainbow
Oct 3, 2015

While all this was happening - finding a new home for Serena, family vacations, work, and a complete house remodel - I was still dealing with ever worsening health problems. The swelling in my eyes due to allergies was so bad it was impairing my ability to do most things. Everything was blurry, like looking through water, so I couldn't read, watching TV was more like hearing it, drive, and I was pretty much a hot mess. With this also comes more Dr. specialists, higher co-pays and more testing. And I'd lost my medical grant in May so all this was now entirely on my shoulders. Nearly $700 in prescriptions and $1000 Dr. Co-pays in June alone.

The trip to Breckenridge was amazing, but I was so miserable (eyes and sight can ruin everything) it was hard to stay positive about the "beautiful" and "peaceful" place meant to be a respite I couldn't see and just found it frustrating. I couldn't go anywhere alone. I couldn't take hikes or walks. I couldn't see the amazingly beautiful things surrounding me. It was all a blur.

I started back to work in August and found my stamina at an all-time low; even worse than last year. 3-4 hours a day was all I could handle for a while, slowly building my strength back up. However, just when I thought the GVHD was retreating, the smoke from the west coast forest fires settled in my lungs and gave me pneumonia. I was out for a week and did my best to do some work from home, but that was silly.

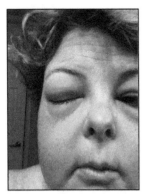

So for the months of August and September I was plagued by swollen, allergy eyes that made my vision blurry and required my first set of glasses ever. I was retaining water from the Prednisone making me very puffy and miserable. The rash/hives on my back, chest, and back was the most itchy, irritating thing ever. My mouth is ridiculously dry all the time and my eyes are so dry I have to put drops in nearly every 30 minutes - this was after 3 trips to eye docs and going through 2 prescriptions and an eye drop steroid that just made things worse. Prednisone also made me moody, depressed, and wired so sleep was elusive. I need sleep to recover but can't sleep so I wasn't getting much better.

The rainbow shining over this storm is my work. I love it and the people I'm working with and am feeling very productive. My endurance has really improved and I'm putting in full days again. Thank goodness because we'd be in real trouble if I had to quit for any reason. My medical bills are close to $1500 a month, that's with insurance, and all the new carpet, flooring, and furnishings put us out close to $20,000. We're getting by every month, but the extra payments are really scary to us.

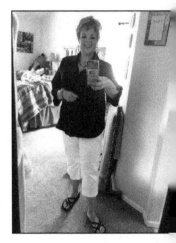

So Joe is taking on more side work and I started selling Mary Kay with my mother-in-law to help ease the financial burden. My sister also set up a GoFundMe account in the hopes our family and friends might help us out with the unintended consequence of being a survivor and having extraordinary and unique situations that are making life hard.

Angela - We love you and will give what we can!!!
Jennifer - You've already given so much of your love and time and prayers and home and meals. We're fortunate to know you and love you too!

Short and Sweet...ish
Oct 6, 2015

So, I was leaving the pharmacy having just spent $400 on one prescription, the one I must take forever, and started crying. It was another bill we can't pay. And add it to the other expenses and the ones yet to come, I just couldn't help but feel hopeless. Getting in the car, John noticed my sadness and quickly said, "God will provide". Giving him a big hug and thanking God for him, I took a deep breath and pulled myself together, saying a little prayer that I didn't really believe would come true. But then I was reminded who was the boss.

I headed to the liquor store to find a way to let this one melt off. What could a little wine hurt? As I was checking out I noticed the scratch tickets and decided to blow $10 on 2 tickets: one for me and one for John. I never do this and felt stupid spending money when I should be saving every last dime. But two minutes later I'd just scratched a ticket for $500!!!!!!!! I've NEVER won more than $2 on a scratch before. God does provide and then some. You should have seen my victory dance and victory whoop in the car. I'm POSITIVE it embarrassed John completely, but he was smiling too. And it was a good thing I'll never forget.

But then I was sad again. I wanted to save up to get John a real "adult" bedroom set: bed with more than just a mattress, a nice dresser, a night stand, and a lamp and some storage. Something he deserves and will only really have for 2 more years before he leaves for college. That $500 would make a good dent in that. But reality and responsibility set in. I am so tired of John's needs coming after mine: He should always come first. That's just not fair. But again, my needs come first, and it makes me wilt to think I can't give him these things.

So I felt prideful before, and never wanted to ask because I didn't want people to know how really bad off we are. And largely because I didn't want to appear weak. But I'm not afraid anymore. If God will respond like he did today, then surly asking for help is not a bad, selfish, weak thing to do. We NEED HELP. Our bills are taking over and we are really scared.

My sister set up a GoFundMe.com account hoping people will help us fend off the bills we can't handle. Please either donate or share it, send it on, whatever. I have known since the beginning the amazing angel team and support system we have, and we need them to help us out again. Joe and John have gone through so much, and Joe has worked so hard to give us a good life, and I feel incredibly guilty that it's all being dumped into me.

Please go to the account and make a donation or share it with others. As you all know, we don't ask for much, but I'm asking now. Please help us.

Honesty
Feb 23, 2016

If you ask me how I'm doing, you'll probably hear "I'm good." If you ask me how I'm feeling, you'll hear "I'm good". And then there's the less positive "I'm doing the best I can with what I've got," or "Things could be worse," or "Some days are better than others." Here's the truth. I'm miserable. My joints, muscles, and bones ache and hurt all the time in spite of stretching and mild exercise. My eyes are swollen and puffy and although I have "20/20 vision", I probably shouldn't be driving. My eyes are either so puffy they make my vision blurry, like looking through someone else's glasses and saying, "oh my God that's bad", or so irritated and dry I feel like gouging them out. Either way, vision is a huge issue. I go through so many eye drops I should buy stock in Bausch and Lomb. And not having your eyes makes everything 200% harder than it needs to be. Think about it. Reading and responding to emails. Hard. Looking at data. Hard. Putting together a presentation. Hard. Reading texts. Hard. And think about how much moving air we're exposed to through the day, AC, heat, car heaters or AC, wind, fans, etc. ALL of which dry my eyes out so fast they hurt. I have headaches. My stomach is upset all the time. Living with these things every day is getting real old, real fast.

I've lost so much. We had to give up our cat because of the suspicion I was allergic. We spent tens of thousands of dollars updating the house with new carpet, flooring, furniture, and vent cleaning. I've lost the ability to be in the sun with the threat of a GVHD breakout, which makes all this worse with skin rashes, diarrhea, and severe fatigue. Not to mention all the get-togethers, celebrations, parties, and other events that I've had to miss or reschedule. I've lost people. And as the weather gets nice, I am reminded I have to cover up and avoid the sun at all costs. And Time. So much time wasted in the car on the way to and from appointments, in the hospital, waiting in Dr. offices, waiting in line for prescriptions, taken by not being able to see or function for one reason or another.

"Good" is all relative. My idea of good is: I woke up today. I can walk and run (at least that's what I call it - John thinks I'm walking). I have all my limbs and no paralysis. I have a son I don't deserve that has been witness to this for 2 years. And now he has to watch me suffer through all this again and can't do anything to help. Joe is a saint but doesn't know what to do either. How could he? He gives great hugs, is positive, and does the best he can to be attentive. I have amazing parents who continue to walk this walk with me, as much as they can. My sister donor is great. All my friends and coworkers and everyone who thinks about or prays for me don't know it, but they make my life worth trying.

I've looked high and low for support groups, of which there are none. I'll travel for trials. I am using "serum tears" made from my own blood cells in an effort to reduce the dry eye issue. I am exposing myself to a chemo treatment once a month to "maintain" some humanity. I've been on a cleanse for 4 weeks that doesn't seem to be making any progress. $200 I'll never get back. I've tried "cupping", massage, meditation, edibles, cannabis oil, drinking and not drinking, healthy diets, protein shakes, naturalistic doctors that gave me products that made me suicidal - yeah, that was fun, hot and cold compresses, so many prescriptions that doctors don't have anything else to try.

One thing that helped, ironically, was becoming a Mary Kay consultant. Being able to dive into making that a success has been a blessing. I've been able to use my past experiences to use social media to promote and sell, to create ways to get the product to people, and still have a "life". One of the best things is that I've been able to reconnect with people I haven't talked to in years. I don't do parties because I don't believe in the obligation it puts on people, but I love open houses and demonstrations. It's my way of seeing people again, after two years of partial seclusion, so please come if you get an invite. It really is more about hosting you and catching up and reconnecting and not the sale. But that all being said, it doesn't make my life easier; it's one more thing to live for.

So, I'm not in the mood to sugar coat this for anyone. You may see me as a strong woman who won and is winning a terrible battle, but I see a person who is suffering. I am faking it til' I make it. That's all there is to it. This is HARD. And some days are better than others. Unfortunately, most days lately have been on the hard side. It's hard to swallow, but I may be as good as I'm ever going to get, and that's just depressing. So tomorrow I'll fight through the day, I'll be "good", and I'll be a semi-productive person. My hope is to someday feel human again. Until then, smile, nod, and say "ok"!

Kari - *Not sure what to say besides we all love u and I'll keep praying my dear sweet, strong friend!! So sorry all this BS is happening!!! Thank you for your real, transparent, honest post!* ♡

Angela - *I hate hearing this but need to. I take for granted the time we do get to spend together shooting guns or at the casino and I shouldn't. I cherish the fun times we have had together and the many yet to come. I wish I had the right words to say but I'm a freaking math teacher and suck at this. We pray for you often and think of you always.*

Gail - *You certainly put our lives into a different perspective. When we think we're having a bad day we have no idea what a bad day really is. Thanks for helping so many of us stop and smell the roses. We love you and will continue to pray for day when you'll feel better.*

Margaret - *I am sorry, Jenn and I truly look forward to the day that all of this is behind you. You did not deserve any of this, but you DO deserve a life free of the complications of cancer. Better days ahead my friend.*

Todd - *You don't deserve this is right. I don't have the words either, even as a wordy guy. But there's great irony in that your suffering has taught so many others a level of perspective unknown otherwise. I'm sorry for you my lady. I thank you for teaching me so much. I'm a believer in that God will not give anyone more than they can handle. You are obviously the strongest of us. (If ever there was any doubt.)*

Rex - *You will always be my JENNIFER ANN in heart & soul ... nothing can/will ever change that. My prayers are not a pious addition to things we would've done anyway ... IT IS A FORCE allowing things to happen which could NOT have occurred without it! Love ya now & forever, your prayerful Daddy*

Chapter 8

Running on Empty

Here we go again and a little bit of desperation
Mar 7, 2016

After my last Rituxan (mild chemo for the GVHD) treatment in January, I felt good for a week or two and then was feeling close to good when things got worse again. I look great. I function well enough for most people not to notice. And my pain, suffering, hell is mine alone to fight. I never thought I would say it, but I'm feeling broken. I'm back in treatment again and don't see a point. A waste of 6 hours of my

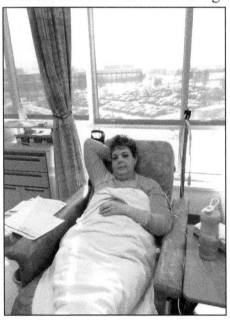

day I'll never get back. There is no time of any day I feel me. None. Closing my eyes is the closest thing I have, and the reality of where that leads is frightening. I don't like waking up knowing I have a fight in front of me and realizing that's probably my reality from now on. Depressing. I am not as strong as you all think. I know the "fake it till you make it" isn't working anymore. I can't hide my squinting and winking eyes. The pain in my scrunched-up forehead. My gaps for words. I'm scared my instructional and leadership experience will never be shared and all I want is to pass on what I know. To help people see their potential from my lens and help them reach it. I've been successful so far with that, but now I'm scared because people are holding me back and I'm not sure how much time I have.

And today in treatment I felt the hopelessness from the nurses too. They couldn't find a vein. They collapsed 2. The one they found for 4 hours of treatment ended up "blowing" somewhere in the drip and unloaded Rituxan into my entire arm and tissues, not just the intended vein. I had to see a specialist to see what to do. Can I survive the Rituxan "spill" into my body or will it create new hurdles? No one knows.

What I HATE IS BEING SEEN AS WEAK BECAUSE I HAVE A SETBACK. A label. Something to define me and ultimately use against me. I am not a victim. Never have been. I've been blessed beyond glory. And I hate ignorance and failure to have grace.

It is what it is.

Gail - Sad to hear the latest news. No words will help. All I can say is I care and will ask God for you to see some hope. Love, Gail

Steph - Oh my love......I'm here. Stay in your brave fight. It's very unfair, but you are such a champion. I love you

Rex - Jennifer - Honey, I'm feeling worse FOR YOU now than that when u were in hospital on the chemo treatments & lugging around your IV pole...not necessarily feeling hopeless but helpless & feeling your confusion, frustration, anxiety & desperate state of mind. You're always in our minds & prayers! This damn insidious disease is hell-on-earth not only 4 u but all those who suffer. My heart bleeds for you. Please O' Lord † give to me all of Jennifer's pain, suffering, anxiety & relieve her of this hellacious burden. Your loving Father

Rene - This makes me so sad. I pray God will carry you through this storm. You are loved by so many.

Round 2
Mar 25, 2016

This GVHD is the bane of all existence. I have never felt so dehumanized, and that's saying a lot. However, this past week I've been doing a LOT of research and have discovered that things could be SO MUCH WORSE, and I have nothing to complain about. But that doesn't lessen the impact I feel on a daily basis. GVHD is a system disorder where my immune system identifies my transplanted stem cells as the enemy and starts a war that can show symptoms in various body systems. The most common are the gut and intestines, skin, eyes, liver, kidneys, lungs, and other soft tissues. In my case I have level 4 (the most severe) eye GVHD. Thankfully the rest of my systems are behaving as they should with the occasional mild reaction. The worst thing about this is that most days I look really good and healthy and am functioning at a high level even though I am miserable on the inside. I am a prisoner in my own body. And people see me and figure I'm doing pretty well and I'm miserable. The eye symptoms have 4 major characteristics: dry/irritated or burning/stinging (puffy or red whites), blurred vision (like looking through a windshield with broken wiper blades or looking through a fish tank or someone else's prescription eyeglasses), goobers that float in my eyes and feel like needles, and light sensitivity. I have all of these, usually not all at the same time, but there's always one that is prominent for that day. I wake up daily wondering what I'm going to have to deal with today. This week it's been extremely blurry eyes and burning/stinging pain.

So, I'm beginning round two of the "Chemo" Rituxan. I'll have 3 more 5-hour treatments that are supposed to settle this internal battle down and bring me back to a more livable and happy quality of life. The good news is that it really doesn't hurt or have any side effects other than being tired. And bruising from the needles. No big deal.

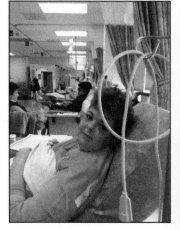

Last week I went to the Allergist to rule out, or in, allergies that may be exacerbating my swollen eyes. The good news is that I'm officially not allergic to anything other than cats, which we knew. That means all the food allergies I had BEFORE the transplant are gone! Simply amazing is all I can say. It also means I don't have to worry about my dog, Sydney, or her bringing in molds or fungus or weeds or pollen. Woohoo!! We are however going back to a "cleaner" way of life again. Not that we were ever really dirty, but we're going to pay more attention to keeping things clean and not let dishes sit in the sink, or piles of dirty laundry pile up, and not let Sydney up on our beds or couches. I'm not sure that last part will ever take hold...Sydney is just too much of a couch dog. And besides, who's going to keep her off when we're not here?

Hope is a wonderful thing. The best of things. - Andy Dufrane, The Shawshank Redemption

h"ALL"elujah and Hope
Mar 25, 2016

So, after nearly two years, I am finally getting some information that will save me and my family. I've been treading water expecting someone with a lifeboat to rescue me and help us navigate this thing called recovery. I've been wondering where all the alternative medicine people are, and the nutritionists, and the support groups, and the assistance....it wasn't anywhere. It was like I had to know the questions to ask to get answers, but who knows the questions to ask when you don't know? See where I'm going with this? I didn't have anyone to hold my hand and help me with finances, or therapies, or appointments, or anything. I kept hearing I needed to go to a counselor, well duh, but where's that? "Get in a group." Really? And where will I find that? I even had a person from the Leukemia Society ask me if I wanted to start my own group?!?! Ah, NO THANK YOU. I have enough on my plate right now.

So, as I'm getting my 3rd treatment, a very nice social worker approached me and asked how I was doing. She started asking me how my recovery was coming and, in a matter of about 5 minutes, she opened the world to me. She gave me a BOOK of everything cancer, arranged by specific cancers, treatments, support groups, travel assistance, financial assistance, non-conventional therapies, and on and on and on to the point of being overwhelming in the other direction. TOO MUCH INFORMATION!! But holy cow. I am SO hopeful!

And then my sister-in-law sorted through the myriad of information on the web using her medical list-serves and studies and such and sent me a condensed list of information that made my heart happy. It grew three sizes that day! Finally, information that was reliable, valuable, and pertinent to me and my family.

And THEN I found a Leukemia/Lymphoma Society Conference on April 16th in Denver! I invited the whole family and can't wait to go meet other people in the same place we are as a family. What a terrific thing for my son who I know doesn't connect to anyone and is very alone in his experience. Maybe he'll find someone to talk and relate to. And Joe needs someone too. I'm hoping there will be spouses he can hook up with.

And the bestest thing ever? A national conference in Chicago at the end of April for Ocular GVHD!!! What? That's exactly what I have, and it has sessions for caregivers and family, and intro on GVHD and fatigue and lack of sleep and side-effects and on and on. Joe and John are going with me to this God-Sent opportunity and I haven't felt this hopeful in over a year.

I keep thinking, where was this when I needed it on the days I felt so hopeless? Maybe I needed all this time to be ready to receive the information. Or maybe my family wasn't ready yet. Whatever the reason, I am headed into a new age of information and assistance and hopefully I won't feel so alone anymore.

One more treatment, a local conference, and a national conference and I'm feeling like I scored the lottery.

Gail - You made my day. I'm so happy and proud of you. Love, Gail
Kari - Woo hoo!!! Great news!

Location, location, location
Mar 25, 2016

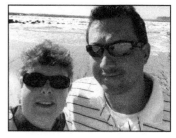

I've been in San Diego for 3 days and am a new woman. I know that after 3 treatments I should expect a certain amount of improvement, but my eyes are back to NORMAL! Yes, I said NORMAL! I think it has everything to do with the moisture in the air. This is amazing. I can see! I haven't excessively needed my drops or timeouts or glasses. It's wonderful. And it makes me think about my future.

What's next for me? Is Colorado a place that is making my life more difficult because it is so dry? Do I need to consider another place, like San Diego, or Florida, with more humidity, that would make all this go away? I don't have that answer. I already have humidifiers at home and work, but they don't seem to be helping the way this natural humidity does.

And being an educator, I should be able to find a job anywhere, right? Joe works for the state patrol and all states have one of those, right? And there's AVID in Hawaii! But Colorado is home. Always has been and all my family is here. I need 4 seasons and the mountains.

They have these contact lenses (Prose or Sclera) that have a pool of moisture in them that I'll learn about at the conferences. I've been trying for a year to get things OUT of my eyes, and now they want to put something in them?! I'll try anything. I'm even looking into trials to see what else might be of help. Interestingly enough, many of the medications and treatments I'm on are still in the "trial" process. The Rituxan (chemo for GVHD) treatment - trial; Sirolimus (for the ALL Ph+) - trial; the serum tears - trial. The newest immunotherapy treatments are simply miraculous and not nearly as dangerous or harmful as chemo or radiation. We're definitely in a new age of practicing medicine.

Anyone want to come to the conference on April 16th? Let me know!

Rex - *Honey ... Your health & well-being is far, far more important than where u choose to live. It's a very mobile society & our fam can always get together easily ... flights go anywhere anytime anymore. YES, we are a close-knit group but our primary concern is that u will be HAPPY & CONTENT & find a new "NORMAL"! If humidity will do the trick ... Then go for it. Perhaps u can take a family vacation & try out the conditions in Florida & San Diego (again) just to confirm that the humidity does indeed help. If contact lens will do the job ... Then try them too. Pull out all the stops*

Gail - Wow. It's so good to hear you had three good days. I would love to hear more about the contacts. I am still asking around about the book. I have gotten amazing response from people. Just don't have a real clear direction. Happy Easter
Kathy - Exciting possibilities and good advice from your dad!

Chapter 9

The Open Road

Not Alone!
Mar 27, 2016

As I mentioned in an earlier post, several posts, I have felt very alone the past two years. I've been on my own to sort through reliable and unreliable websites, organizations, articles, offers, and programs. I've been begging for a lifeline to ANYONE that I could talk to that might understand what I am going through. A support group would have been great, but there isn't one. And when I asked, they asked me to start one. (Exactly where would you like me to start with that? - That's the whole problem.) And health professionals do a TERRIBLE job of helping. They're in their own reality and because of HIPAA laws, can't even give my contact information to someone else going through similar things, even if it's 'OK' with me. Lost. Alone.

Don't get me wrong. I have an incredible support system of family, friends, acquaintances, and perfect strangers all doing, and praying, and thinking, for and about me and my family. I'm blessed beyond words that way. And I'm not "alone". Not really. But when you lay it all out there and tell people how you feel, and all they can do is nod their head and try to understand but how can they possibly, the feeling is so empty. I know how much they really care and would do anything to help me deal, but I still feel shallow and hollow.

But that's changed. That Cancer Book I got has opened a whole new world. It's overwhelming how much information is in it, but I'm going through it slowly and finding things that will and won't help. Among them was through the Leukemia and Lymphoma Society and they set me up with a fellow survivor that I can talk to. Brian. His blessed, hopeful, understanding, lifesaving name is Brian. And in just the few days we've emailed and texted, I feel like a new world has opened. He has seen everything I have. He has been through the chemo and radiation and a stem cell transplant and chronic GVHD. He knows. He's had the advantage of having a support group of people since he was in transplant, but I'm so great with that. He can and is showing me a new world of Jennifer Specific supports that only I can understand are so critical to my recovery. I have a purpose again. Instead of asking why bother get through another day, I am looking forward to the day and the next. Looking at the positives again, like even though my eyes are blurry today, it could get better and at least they don't hurt too.

I say it over and over again and I really mean it. Things could be so much worse. I feel fortunate that I haven't been in Brian's shoes. I have my own path to travel and I'm guessing that I needed to be right here in this place to value the gift I've been given.

Rex - I kinda/sorta know how u relate to your supportive guy "Brian"...as a long time recovering alcoholic the past 22 years "THANX" to sooo many people in all walks of my life...I have discovered the only real & genuine people that can fully understand my condition, treatment & recovery are those that are themselves "recovering alcoholics"...be it thru AA, close friends & of course my fam. Be that as it may, having been thru your own hell in battling leukemia & now this GVHD aftermath crap...it warms my heart to know that someone like Brian can relate & share your common realities. We all have your own personal demons to deal with! God bless both of you. Maybe you don't fully "get it" yet but you have just started your own SUPPORT GROUP...similar to me being close to my AA sponsor & confidant. Love ya now & forever, Dad p.s. We are never really "ALONE" ya know...when we fully understand how your "HIGHER POWER" can fit into your lives, feel your pain, understand your soulful prayers...Guess who is always listening? †

Gail - What great news. I'll pray for Brian your new angel also. ☺

Melissa - There's my girl.

153

Getting Back in the Saddle
Apr 8, 2016

Coming up on my 2-year transplant birthday I am at odds with everything. There are so many things going on and I've felt very broken. I'm taking small steps to find myself again, including acupuncture. I found someone that listens and has literally opened me back up again. My body has been so toxic it doesn't know even how to take a deep breath and relax or let things go. The acupuncture has been exhausting but I believe it's working. I've found a new mindfulness that feels more like me.

Physically I'm feeling better too. Although I still wake up daily with eye issues (blurry, stinging pain, dry, irritated), it's better than it's been. I think the Chemo treatments have been shutting down the GVHD and I am starting to heal. That's good. And Spring Break has given me the time to shut out the things that are externally toxic. Things like adults acting like children. Grow up. The silent treatment is stupid. Avoiding eye contact is middle school. Keeping secrets, gossip, and cliques are ridiculous. Really? I'm surprised I don't get more, "check yes or no" emails.

It's funny how getting things done, especially for women, I think, can clear the mind too. I got taxes done, paid bills, and got a jump start on stuff outside. Of course, that just makes my list longer but having purpose is important. I needed to adjust my focus back to me and not the things happening around me. I'm happier that way.

And no one has any idea what I have, am, or will go through. I have to remember that other peoples' judgement is irrelevant. It's interesting how so many things are really just the same now as they were before cancer. It's just my new "thing" to deal with, just like everyone else.

<u>Rex</u> - Jenn - Your continued wonderful understanding of your current condition(s) is sooooo very awe inspiring ... If only the whole world could see the beauty of what surviving horrendous & traumatic health issues looks like thru your vision of life & "DEALING" w/ the day-to-day reality of living life on life's terms! Just keep on truckin' honey. 👍 🌸 Love ya, Dad

Answers
May 28, 2016

At the end of April, we (Joe, John, and I) went to Chicago to attend a Bone Marrow Transplant Conference for survivors and caregivers. IT WAS AMAZING. They had sessions on everything I've been desperate to find. Dealing with insomnia, dealing with fatigue, GVHD of the eyes (this is what I have) and every other GVHD area as well (gut, mouth, skin, lungs, organs). We met some really incredible people and got a lot of answers and "a-ha" moments. I think it was very eye-opening, especially for the boys. They got to see people like me and realize I'm not doing things on purpose, like forgetting conversations or being tired or needing help with stuff I used to be able to do without blinking an eye. That when I ask for help it's because I either can't do it at all or I really need help, not because I'm lazy or trying to punish anyone. We all saw that as bad as I think I have it some days, my worst days are many people's dream day. We are VERY lucky and blessed to be where we are now. My symptoms, as much as they stink, could be SO MUCH WORSE. I couldn't believe how really bad it could get. Living in my own little world I didn't realize most people don't return to work...ever...and I just finished my 2nd full year of work. Some people get the skin GVHD so bad their skin gets tight and they can't move their limbs and have painful hives all over their body. And so many people are constantly sick with infections or colds, or pneumonia. Joe was able to spend time with a group of caregivers, just like himself, with a spouse who has/had leukemia. He met someone who lives just south of us in Castle Rock and has talked to him a couple times since the conference. I also met my people and was so relieved to get to know some of them. There were at least 5 people who not only had ALL like I did, they also had the fearsome and dreadful PH+ chromosome diagnosis. Back in the day, less than 10 years ago, the PH+ strand was a certain death sentence. But now with the new immuno-therapies being developed, they can cure it completely. It's mind blowing to think about.

I can't wait to take all the stuff I brought back with me to my BMT Docs. They were the ones that told me about the conference and encouraged me to go. And they want a full report at my next appointment. I'm excited to show them all the(new therapies and medicines and treatments that are available. And to give them the handouts from all the sessions so they can help others like me. It feels good to know that I can help someone I don't even know who is suffering like I did/do just by attending a conference and bringing back the knowledge.

What I learned for myself is that I am remarkable. I often struggle with sleep and fatigue, and my eyes are very annoying most days, but I've got it easy. I also found out that the GVHD may get better with time, but chances are I'll have this forever in one form or degree or another. That could be depressing to some and honestly not what I wanted to hear, but I can live with it. I've learned how to cope with dry eyes and get by with little sleep and I'm ok with that.

Rex - *We're sooooo happy u & Joe & John were able to go as a fam unit & discover together 1st hand the many effects & treatments of GRAFT VERSUS HOST DISEASE. It will become an increasingly valuable tool as time as goes on to be able to openly share that experience & knowledge. U R a gift to all that know the "WARRIOR" in U & can share your passion & thirst to gain more knowledge about this whole horrible experience & your battle(s) the past 2 1/2 yrs. Hope U can document all this in a publication so the entire world will be able to better understand the before, during & after trials & tribulations of this insidious cancer called LEUKEMIA PH+ ... I love your savvy explanation of this Conference in Chicago. Thanx 4 sharing. Love, Dad*
Gail - *Thanks for sharing. We can now share with other people we meet and help them to realize their options and hope. Love you. God is so good.*

Reality
May 28, 2016

I have decided there is no such thing as reality. It's all about perception. Reality forces a description. Perception is emotion. And everyone's perception is their own reality. For example, if you get a "D" on a test that you were sure you were going to fail, your perception is "Yes!" But reality is you did less than average and barely passed. And I once told John that the difference between negativity and reality is experience. Pretty brilliant if you ask me. But lately my perception, reality, and experience have not aligned at all. That's what cancer does. It mixes everything up and makes life unpredictable based on anything. Emotion, behavior, action, ability, preference, outcome...you name it.

I find myself weighing things differently now. And I am constantly spun in 90 different directions at a moments' notice. A few weeks ago, I cursed my eyes. Today my eyes are great (no stinging, blurred vision, pain, and only a few drops), but I wiped myself out this past weekend doing yard work - because I could and haven't been able to in three years - and now my right arm rotator cuff is out of action. I mean I can't move it. In a sling with a rotation of heat and cold. I can't turn over in bed and I'm doing everything with my left hand. I mean, really? Reality is I shouldn't have pushed myself so hard. Perception is I was so freaking happy I didn't even realize I was pushing. Until I woke up the next day not being able to move my arm. I wouldn't change a thing. Regaining something I love and dealing with the temporary aftermath of a hurt wing for a week or so was and is worth it. That's perception vs. reality.

But I also deal with 180-degree swings of despair and joy. Some days I am SO ok checking out and not dealing with anything. I mean severe depression and overwhelming negativity that is consuming and my full reality. I don't want to be here feeling anything. I don't want to sleep or be awake or be. Period. I am done.

But other days I am consumed with simple joys. Like a birds' nest under my deck with two birdies and a momma and poppa that will defend their babies. Or a Monarch butterfly that doesn't just float by (I believe they're spirits of people I love and rejoice at seeing one because it's visiting me), but land on my tree branch and just hang out. That's glorious to me.

And I'm trying to find a way to be more level with everything. Acupuncture, Mindfulness classes and meditation, trying to separate/change reality from perception, finding peace. It's not working. Lol. Yesterday I was desperately sad. Today a little more hopeful. Tomorrow? We shall see I guess. But I have plans for the future and that means everything.

Karen - Beautifully stated. I can sympathize with you with my Ostomy. Not used to have all these feelings. Up down and around!!

Strength
May 29, 2016

Since the very beginning of this chapter in my life, people have said all kinds of things about strength. How strong I am. That I'm a fighter. That Leukemia doesn't have a chance. Gave me boxing gloves. That I inspire, amaze, bewilder, create hope and am a miracle. I never wanted this or to be any of those things. I woke up in the morning, went through all sorts of treatments, suffered unbelievable evil, and lived through it. That's all. I lived. But I also had faith. I woke up every morning thankful to wake up. I'd look at the mountains or the trees outside my hospital window and just be there. I'd pray. I'd find something to be thankful for. And I thank Eric, one of my nurses, for giving me that advice. Find something every day that you can be thankful for. Find your blessings. Look for the good. And there were definitely days that I really struggled to find any good in anything. Some days it was a simple thing like finishing a crossword puzzle. I guess when I think about it, most of the gifts were small things. A blood test that showed improvement. Not feeling nauseated. Getting the feeling back in my fingers. A sunrise. My family and visitors. The blankets my mom made me. The Broncos winning. Every test that came back negative...or positive...however you want to look at it. Knowing Dr. Hyde was a true practitioner of medicine and took my case personally.

And as I started to find a little more normalcy once going home, even then it was simple things. Like going to the bathroom without having a "hat" in the bowl. Taking a shower without using anti-bacterial soap that dried out my skin. Not having to flush my PICC line or wear a sleeve over it in the shower. Ahhhhh, the freedom you can't imagine unless you have experienced it. Sleeping in my own bed, all night, without interruptions every 2-4 hours. Hugging people without them wearing a mask, gloves, or a gown. Making my own food. Driving. Taking one less prescription because I didn't need it anymore. Having a glass of wine. Wearing real clothes, not just pajamas or sweats. Not breathing hospital air.

Being a "survivor" is something I refuse to call myself. I didn't survive. I woke up, every day, and just did what was thrown at me. I had no control over anything my body was doing. We all have managed to live through one thing or another. And saying I'm a survivor makes me feel like I am a victim, and I **refuse to be a victim**. I had a choice, every day, to pick the day I wanted to have. I could be happy I woke up, or pissed off because I woke up. I could blame someone, or realize things just happen. I could be an "awful-izer" or a "real-izer". I often wonder how I did make it. I mean, I'm a very competitive person, but the game I was playing didn't have any rules. My opponent was invisible. I couldn't practice, I didn't know the skills involved, there wasn't a game plan, and I didn't know how to score. And it seemed that once I figured out the game, I'd get called for a penalty and have to find a new strategy. But somehow, I won. I am winning. And I've been wondering why. Where does this "strength" come from?

And then this week it occurred to me that my strength comes from my faith. My God carried me when I couldn't carry myself. Like footsteps in the sand, it was then that he carried me. And although I felt closer to God during my fight than I ever have before, I didn't see that he wasn't just with me, he was in me, fighting for me, and giving me his strength. Through him, ALL things are possible. Ironic that ALL is the name of my cancer.

So, I've changed how I feel about being called strong. Hearing that I'm an inspiration. Being a fighter. What people are seeing is God moving, acting, and living through me. I couldn't ask for anything better than that. To know that I am living a good life. And whether you believe in a higher power or not, I didn't do this through my own strength and will. There was another power involved that sustained me when I couldn't do it myself. I am thankful for that and am choosing to allow that strength to run through me and guide me and hope that others will continue to see me as a fighter.

But that's not all. I was also filled with the strength of every person who sent positive thoughts, prayed for me, and supported me and my family. That is so powerful. I am living because I had a team of fighters behind me that refused to let us lose. It is said that God only gives you what you can handle...well I thank him for sharing his strength and putting all the people in my life that kept my battle a win-able one. I always said that but didn't really get it until now. I can't, didn't and won't do this without my angel team. The fight goes on and I am thankful.

Mom - Maybe that's a name for your book -I Lived or I am Living. Such beautiful thoughts, Jenn. Loving you, Mom

Rex - Wonderful Babe 👊 🍪: You've come a very long way on your journey in more ways than one. You have given me the gift of FAITH in GOD 🔒 🍪 that I didn't realize was in me... Now I do & it feels great! Thank you, Jennifer, cuz your father has become a new guy & I like him. Finally, after 70 years, I have found the "tools" to openly live, love & share my faith. God bless, Dad †

Gail - This is so powerful. Thanks for sharing. As you said all things are possible through God if we will let him work within us.

Rene - I am so touched by your testimony of faith. It was worded so perfectly. God has not only carried you through but given you the wonderful gift of being able to express your feelings. I am so glad things are going well for you.

No News is Good News
Jul 17, 2016

This has been a remarkable summer to say the least. I am experiencing things for the first time since I was sick and LOVING IT! My "new" normal is finally starting to look like my "old" normal a lot. And I'm totally taking advantage of every opportunity I have been given to live again. And I'm doing them without fear of

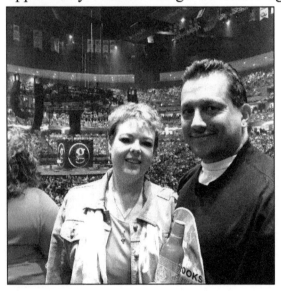

getting or catching something. Fear is a terrible thing, but I've turned it into opportunity and just use precautions when doing something that has been problematic in the past. I use sunscreen, wear hats and gloves, stay out of the sun, take frequent breaks, use bacterial soap and hand sanitizer, and stay hydrated. I love that I can wake up and choose the activity I want to do that day without the restrictions in the past. It's fun to decide "what do I want to do today?" Here are some "firsts" that finally made me feel like me again:

* Garth Brooks Concert!
* Went camping
* Went fishing - still have yet to catch anything other than weeds but I'm doing it
* Went boating
* Gardening - finally planting, pruning, watering, deadheading - it's so freeing and gives me satisfaction of accomplishment
* Spending time on my patios - front and back - just being

* Landscaping projects that have irritated me for a long time
* Having friends over around the fire pit
* Sit on my deck for extended periods of time
* Quality time with John
* Watched sunsets outside and not from a window
* I'm listening to the birds, watching them build nests and hatch eggs, setting up hummingbird feeders, and just sitting to experience it
* Doing projects around the house that I didn't have the strength or energy to do before - cleaning out my closet for example

I've been busy and not busy at the same time. Nothing feels rushed or emergent. And I have two more weeks to make the most of summer. Hmmmmm...I wonder what I'll do?? :-)

Eldon - Good for you Jennifer. God has blessed you and your and your family. I can't think of anybody more deserving. Your struggle and success will always be a strong reminder for me to live each day to the fullest. Take care and enjoy his blessing.

Best Seller?
Jul 21, 2016

So, I'm doing it. I've decided to write a book. Well, I've already written it here and in my journals throughout my experience, but I'm doing it. I've transcribed 65 pages so far and that barely gets me through October the first year. I thought it would be easy just cutting and pasting what I'd already written, but I'm reading it as I go and feel one emotion after another surface or hit me like a brick. And re-reading the amazing comments from people remind me how much I relied on their strength, not mine, to get me through a day. And as I read through the journal entries, memories I didn't write about come back and I realize there are blanks I need to fill in. I'm not leaving anything out, though. It happened, and it was real and if it mattered enough to write about then, it's worth leaving in there now.
I'm writing while I'm in Oncology getting a maintenance treatment, one that takes 5 hours or so every other week. It's a lot of what could be wasted time, but I'm going to use it productively. I always have because it's actually a long stretch of

time that I'm not getting barraged with phone calls or meetings or other things. It's "sit in the chair" quiet time, sorta. I still have to endure the bells and beeping of machines around me letting nurses know treatments are done or lines are "occluded". Sometimes I get a little PTSD with it, but I remind myself I get to go home. And I get A LOT done!

I'm feeling terrific. I'm hoping these maintenance treatments are doing the trick and getting rid of the GVHD. I am only using eye drops a few times a day now instead of a few times and hour. My skin is clear, my stomach isn't upset, and my brain is clear. I'm feeling so good the fears start creeping in. I've always believed that the good is always accompanied by the bad in a natural, cosmic, cycle of balance and life. And so, I wait for the other shoe to drop. I am hoping the changes at work are the low and I'm dealing with that the only way I know how. With a positive outlook. I also believe we always end up where we are supposed to be so why worry? But the "what if's?" still make an appearance and I have to do my best to stop allowing the unknown ruin a perfectly great day.

I have one week of summer left before I have to go back to work in August. I'm not sure how I feel about that. I have done so many things this summer and really feel like I've been able to recoup the energy and passion necessary to work with kids, adult, and adults who act like kids. I don't want this goodness to change. I like the place of contentment and peace I'm in and don't want anything to disrupt it. I want to deal with things as they come, realize I don't have control, I probably didn't create the issue, and it's up to me how I react to it. I'm going to laugh in the face of things that try to interrupt my bubble of goodness and walk away feeling empowered and free.

But back to the book. I hope I can touch just one person, someone newly diagnosed, going through treatment, post care, in remission, caregiver, family member, friend, co-worker, neighbor...anyone who has found themselves in the new world of cancer, or even having been under its curse for years. I felt so incredibly alone my first 2 years not having a group to go to or knowing anyone that could understand MY journey. Everyone's cancer is theirs alone to experience and will take a course completely unique to them. But there are many similarities in the treatments, the emotions, the experiences, the fears, the celebrations that we all need to feel like we're not alone. Not ever. People's thoughts and prayers are always surrounding us with love and strength and the support to take another step, breath, and one day at a time. I hope my words can comfort, heal, support, educate, and inspire when the words are exactly what someone needs to hear at that moment. Sometimes hope is all we have, and I want my words to spread hope.

Steph - *You are beautiful.*
Paula - *Wonderful idea!! I am sure it will be helpful!!!*
Jean - *Thoughts and prayers for your strong spirit in the coming weeks. It's good to hear that you face the days with peace and hope. Keep writing. Your voice makes a difference*

BELIEVE
August 1, 2016

If you've been following my posts, you might notice that I changed the banner at the top to "Believe". If you know me at all, you know I believe in many ways. Whether you're a Tebow fan or not, that season he got us to the playoffs, the chant was "Believe". I did. My son's goldfish, named Tebow, once jumped out of his bowl, was dead and crispy, but came back to life after John put him back in the bowl and started praying. Tebow lived another 2 years. I believe it was a miracle. There is NO WAY that fish should have lived. No joke. I believed in every single one of my students and had the daily battle of helping them believe in themselves. I believed I could beat cancer and I did. And the license plate on my car says "B3LI3V3" (Believe was already taken so I had to improvise). And I have a firm belief in a higher power greater than myself that guides my path and guards my soul. I believe things happen for a reason. I believe we are exactly where we are meant to be. I believe people are dropped into our lives when we need them, and sometimes they fade when we don't. I believe that people are good and act out of positive intention. I believe positive thoughts and prayer really work. I believe in unanswered prayers.

But there have been times when I had a hard time holding my belief in anything. And I'm going to let you into a little secret. About a month ago, I was told my latest test results showed trace amounts of the Leukemia. I was crushed and scared to death. Terrified it was back. I didn't tell anyone other than family because the more people I told, the more real it became. My new Dr., Dr. Hyde retired much to my sadness, said she was not concerned but wanted me to get a second check and moved

163

up the timeframe 2 months. That was alarming to me. Much more emergent than I wanted it to be. I gave the telling and threatening blood sample last week. One whole month of wondering if it was back, trying to move forward like it wasn't, my belief wasn't strong at all. Like I said in my last post, I'm waiting for the shoe to drop because I'm feeling so good. But yesterday I found out it was a false positive! I am still cancer free, thank the Lord. But ironically it has shaken my belief, not strengthened it. I can't explain it, but now I'm on high alert instead of relaxing into a safe place.

Depression has been a daily battle. I've been bullied at work and am having panic attacks about returning this week. I've asked myself "why me?" during the past 8 months and I NEVER did while going through the cancer battle. Cancer happened. I had no control over it. Why not me? I'm not that special. But when it comes to work, I take things very personally. I put my heart and passion into everything I do and when that is questioned, I become defensive. In spite of my accomplishments, I am being held down. And it shakes my belief and confidence to the point of running. I'm actually considering a career change. One that might utilize my background and degrees in Sports Administration and Recreation while counting on my 20 years of education. Let's face it, working with teenagers has given me experience in damage control, character building, de-escalation, problem solving, and leadership and supervision. Skills easily transferred and desired in many careers. But reality has me knowing I'll be returning to work on Tuesday and will have to face my fears and the people who are setting me up to fail.

So, I'm having to take it back to simplicity and believing in me. Believing in my path and my higher power to lead me there. My problem is patience and wanting an answer now. I refuse to be a victim but am having a difficult time finding the strength to resist the easy path of doubt. I still need your positive thoughts and prayers. I BELIEVE that's what helps me get through each day and I don't have the energy to do this on my own. I think I need to be selfish for a little while and pay attention to me. My nutrition, my exercise, my faith, my relationships all need to be first and I think I'll use this new school year to do just that. I'll admit I've been lazy about all those things for one excuse or another, and I think it's time to let the excuses go and take action. I'm going to focus on the things I'm grateful for, the things that I have control over, and my own attitude. As I tell my son, Choose your day. It can be good or bad depending on your choice. So that's what I'm going to do. I'm going to choose my day and hopefully, I will believe I am where I am supposed to be once again.

So That Just Happened
August 25, 2016

Well, I got through my first week of work without students and did everything I could to grin and bear it. I felt very healthy and full of energy and didn't let things, like not having a classroom or office, get me down. I did what I could and left when I couldn't go any further. I also paid more attention to the people who were genuinely interested in me and students and less interested in immature drama. That helped me see who my people are, and who not to associate with or give two shits about. That's really important. Letting people join or leave your circle based on what you need. I don't need doubt or guilt, I don't need to prove anything, I don't need to answer to anyone, and I don't need negative Nancy's. I ended the week with hope in my heart.

I started the week with students unlike ANY week I've ever had in education. As a type A person, my ADD made it necessary to have my room in order, posters up, routines in place, and lesson plans for the first week. For reasons out of my control, NONE of that happened. My new room is a multipurpose room and they were doing registration the week before kids came. So, on the first day, I didn't have tables, chairs, or supplies. I didn't have copies made because I didn't have access to a computer. BC (before cancer) I would have let that ruin everything. But luckily, I'm a kick-ass teacher and had a full week of authentic activities for the students to do while creating a safe, fun, encouraging, positive and team-centered environment. It worked! The kids love me, and I started caring a lot less about who I thought I was supposed to be, and more on who I was. I am a teacher and I should be with students.

Then the hammer came down. On Friday of my first week, which I was so PROUD I had finished smelling like daisy's, I had a Dr. appointment and noticed more drainage and pain in my eye than normal. They said it was pink-eye. After 20 years in education, I KNOW what pinkeye looks and feels like and this wasn't it. I told them that, but they insisted the eye drops would take care of any infection that might be in there. If you've been following me from the beginning, you know what's coming next.

By Saturday morning, my eye was significantly swollen and hurt so bad I couldn't move it. I had Joe take me to the After-Hours care and they gave me a ZPAC. Pretty strong stuff. But my body had a different idea. By Monday it was swollen shut and was giving me a migraine and sinus pain due to the swelling moving into my brain and sinuses. I went back to the Dr. where they promptly put me in a bed and gave me an IV and 2 new antibiotics. The diagnosis was Ocular Cellulitis, an infection of the skin and tissues surrounding the eye, not the eye itself. My vision was fine, my eye was the normal white color, but I looked like I had a black eye. Of course, I was told I had a severe case of it and it would take 10-14 days to clear up, but at least I knew what it was and my instincts, as usual, were right on the money. THIS WAS NOT PINKEYE. Tuesday, there really wasn't much change and I had to call work to tell them I would be out all week. That's what they get for moving me out of a position where I was slightly less exposed to infections and germs into a Petrie dish of funk and filth.

I've been in agony all week. The pain and discomfort at times is torture. I feel like I have glass in my eye. I use ice and heating packs, drops, ibuprofen, and am having a huge dose of couch time watching blurry re-runs of stupid summer shows. Thankfully, good ol' dad saved my sanity and soul and surprised me by coming up on Tuesday just to hang out with me. All of a sudden, things weren't so bad. Even though all he could give me were hugs, which are healing in themselves, at least I wasn't alone. And he didn't feel quite so helpless.

And while I still often cry in the shower or car or on my porch and ask "what did I do?", I am daily reminded that this is just my thing for now. Everyone has their "thing". Stephanie broke her ankle the day before going back to work. HER ANKLE! She's hobbling around in a soft cast, wheelchair, scooter thingy, and crutches with 2nd graders for the first 6-8 weeks of school. Who does that? My buddy Brian, who was diagnosed with the same thing I have, is still so sick after 5 years he hasn't been able to return to work at all and has severe gastro-intestinal issues. Becky's house and truck were totaled...TOTALED...by an ice storm a few weeks ago after getting new windows installed. Tens of thousands of dollars of damage. The new, supposed to be undamageable roof is destroyed, all the siding looks like golf balls, windows broken, trees uprooted. She says it's like a war zone and the appraiser can't get there until this week. Another close friend of mine lost a student, uncle, and cousin within a matter of 24 hours. Who, EVER, has it in them to deal with these things?

So, pray for me, and all the people I talked about above, and each other. Be kind. Show grace and understanding. And be thankful that whatever has you ready to jump off the cliff right now, is probably someone else's wish come true. I have to remind myself that sometimes our worst day is someone else's best day, and to refocus on what I have that is good. "It could be worse" is NOT a poster quote or something to say lightly. I mean it and have that "worse" in mind every time I say it. Sometimes I wish I wasn't dealing with the day I was dealt, but I'd rather have my day than anyone else's because tomorrow I know where I'll wake up and who will be with me and that things can get better.

A New Hope
November 15, 2016

I giggled to myself when I named this chapter because it's the name of a Star Wars movie. But I think it pertains because sometimes I feel like I'm taking on the whole universe against the evil empire. The past few months have been HARD!! I FELT like I was frozen in Carbonite like Han Solo or thrown into the garbage shoot while trying to save the princess only to find it locked with a monster swimming around. Everywhere I turned I faced danger, oppression, and fear. Being in the classroom was dangerous to me and my health, literally life threatening, but I felt like I had no choices and to someone who is as competitive as they come, I refused to give up. I was oppressed by my work and the negative, unkind people surrounding me and I had lost my purpose. I was scared to death of the seemingly dark future ahead, the potential of quitting my job, and no income. This is a petrifying place to be in. And for one of the few times since my diagnosis, I questioned my faith A LOT. I was now asking why? What did I do? And I'm ashamed to say it, but really cursing God. Which also made me feel alone and worthless and hopeless and bad.

And people didn't seem to understand what I had survived and am STILL dealing with and my daily struggle to just get out of bed, let alone go to a job that was literally killing me. Little compassion. Little grace. It has been a rough go. I knew what I needed to do, but knew I needed some sort of income whether it was disability (no guarantee), possible retirement, or a job in education in a different place. I was SO lost, but then God threw me a brick to the head. That's what we call it when the whispers don't work, or we aren't listening, and then God does an intervention and makes things crystal clear. I was being closed minded. I could change my path entirely and go the real-estate route like my dad and sister! I was suddenly so excited

I couldn't stand it. I had a renewed hope and looked into classes, had lunch with Gail (my dear friend), and made some decisions. Now that I knew I could have a future, it was time to act.

And just that one brick literally brought everything, and I mean EVERYTHING, full circle. I decided to give my notice and quit my job. The moment I did that the chains were lifted, and I could breathe again. I would be ok. We would be ok. It was time for a new chapter.

Rex - Jenn - _A NEW BEGINNING ... Is off to a running start! Sometimes when I watch a fly try to keep trying to go out the window screen & all it needs to do is turn around & fly out the open door...seems logical but the fly was just unable to change course. Your making really good well thought out decisions & will undoubtedly land on your feet. I'm excited to sit back & watch your NEW ADVENTURES & a NEW BEGINNING. God bless † Dad_

The Full Circle and A New Chapter
November 16, 2016

I mentioned in my last post how my world was coming around full circle and leading flawlessly into my new chapter. But something happened I NEVER saw coming or even weighed into the picture. A miracle of sorts. It's like God knew, somehow, I'd need this next part to truly heal and have a complete recovery from my entire experience. I know my words won't give it the justice it deserves, but I'll try.
Through a dear friend, I connected with a woman who was diagnosed with the same thing I had, Acute Lymphoblastic Leukemia, and was about to go through the stem cell transplant process. She wanted to know if I would go and talk to her. I couldn't contain my excitement. I was also anxious and scared of the memories that might come back, but my desire to help her as much as I could overcame any feelings of doubt. I would have done ANYTHING to have had someone to talk to that had gone through all this before so I could compare notes. That would have been SO helpful. But we were very alone, secluded for my health, and even though we couldn't do anything about it at the time, I can change that for someone else.

As I drove to the same hospital I was treated in, I was waiting for some overwhelming emotion to take over but was surprised there wasn't much there. I parked like I was anyone visiting someone at the hospital...no history creeping up on me. I went to the gift shop and got some blow-up fake flowers, knowing she couldn't have the real thing around her, and headed up to her room. The funny thing is, in spite of having spent 30 days there myself 2 years earlier, I didn't know where I was going. I spent all my time on the transplant floor and only went through the lobby as I left that last day. This time I was a visitor and not a patient. And it occurred to me that this was what everyone who visited me felt like. The other side of the fence, and it was powerful. They told me her room number and I scanned my Swiss Cheese memories for any recollection or familiarity and found none. So, I headed upstairs. As I stepped off the elevator I didn't recognize anything. It looked fresh and new and light in comparison to the dark, drab, confined halls I remembered. I was thankful for that, in some strange way. I asked a nurse where to go and as we walked to the room, I told her my back-story. She teared up and I'll admit this took me off guard, but I was happy to be there. When we got to the room, she reminded me of the routine I had to go through before going in. This was exactly what I had hoped for. A look into what my family went through every time they visited me from their perspective. And here it was. I washed my hands, put on the yellow gown, found the right sized plastic gloves, and grabbed the flowers.

As I went to open the door, a small spark of "now what? Do I just go in?" occurred to me. I knocked on the door as it happened thousands of times to me but was slightly weird to be the creator and not the recipient and entered the room. Both of us were nervous as we'd never met, but we'd heard a lot about each other, so conversation was easy. And we settled into an amazing conversation with lots of questions, lots of answers, and lots of memories. She asked me about things I had long forgotten, like what did I like to eat, and I really had to search my brain for some answers. Some things I didn't know at all, some things made me giggle. And ALL of it was so revealing to me, opening one onion layer at a time. It was good to be there for her, but it was a blessing for me to see her in the same state I had been in. And I could completely empathize with, honestly relive, what she was going through, and it was NORMAL. Knowing that I was normal was so validating it literally healed parts of me I didn't know were still recovering. Touched places so buried it hurt. And seeped into the cracks of my broken soul, breaking it open and flooding me with joy. It made it real and I found pride and happiness and acceptance of my experience. My life. My struggle. And it felt amazing to be able to share with someone else that what they were feeling is what I felt...exactly the same. Immense fatigue, pain, despair, chills, shakes, no appetite...but it would all get better soon. Slowly, so be patient with yourself, but it's going to be ok.

Then, as the conversation paused for a minute for meds, I laid back in the chair by the window. Just as I thought things couldn't get any more real, I realized I was looking out the window at the exact same scene I had 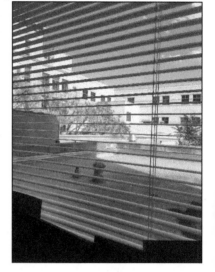 gazed at for 30 days during my transplant. Until that moment I hadn't recognized it, but we were in MY room. My room. My trees. My roof. My sky. I sat there every day watching the trees bloom, and the skies clear and pray and think and cry and suffer. That view, framed by my window, opened the flood gates of emotions I'd been expecting all day. It was a good thing when I noticed her eyes drooping, said my see-you-later's, and made my exit. I thought surely, I'd start bawling any moment and was surprised to find that whatever sadness, anger, doubt, emotion I thought I'd have was replaced by peace. Just peace.

I've wondered for months how this book would end and now it's so clear. I have come full circle. From diagnosis to helping someone just like me. And a new chapter for me with a very unclear but hopeful future. I honestly can't remember the last time I felt this free, but it makes up for every day I felt a prisoner of the cancer, my hospital room, my own home, my body, my circumstance. God did that. He put this together and who would have imagined on January 6, 2014, I'd eventually see more good in this than bad? That I see how so many things I once questioned come together for my good, not my demise. And not just me, but so many people around me. It answered some of my prayers, and I can't argue with that. Words I've said many times are the only way I know how to finish this story.

Hope. Pray. Grace and kindness. Make every day your "someday". Find something every day to be thankful for. BELIEVE.

You never know how STRONG you are until being strong is the only CHOICE you have.

Epilogue

The Next Leg of the Journey

Looking Back
February 2018

I'm not going to lie. It's been a REALLY ROUGH year. After being forced into early retirement October of 2016, I forced myself to see the good. The honest truth of it was I wasn't at all prepared for retirement like most people are. For most, you look forward to retirement, plan for it, wait, think about all the things you want to do, have a countdown, and celebrate the career you had. Not me. I woke up on October 1st and admitted to myself the school district wasn't going to help me. I had to force myself through the agonizing decision to stay in the classroom and risk my life daily, or retire, 10 years too early, and hope God could get me through this too. October 23rd I met with my superintendent and officially resigned. I was really surprised how free I felt immediately after making that decision. I drove home in tears.

I was also terrified. I didn't know what I was going to do. It took me months to actually say the words, "I'm retired". I managed to fill my time with paperwork and such through the start of the year, but still didn't know how I was going to make up for the salary I was now left with. Half. HALF! And I had to cancel things I'd earned through my 20 year career. Cable TV. Subscriptions. Memberships. Things I couldn't afford anymore and I felt robbed. First it was my health, then my normal, and now my career. And my purpose. I woke up every day not knowing what to do. I even tried to bring an American with Disabilities Act case, but the feds didn't feel as though I had a case. If I didn't, I don't know what one would look like.

I was severely depressed and for the first time since my diagnosis, I was asking why me, doubting God, and I couldn't see the good in anything. Nothing. I'd definitely lost me and my happiness. At some point I thought I could start a second career in real estate or focus on Mary Kay or….? I really didn't want to do anything. I was also very angry. Cancer had stolen everything from me. The things I "lived for" through my battle – getting back to my job, getting back to happy, getting back, period – were taken from me.

But I had to find something. Just to wake up with a plan. So I applied at a local fitness center and started working very part time in June. It was great! Being with people who were health centered, meeting up with a personal coach who was cancer certified and really helped me accept me where I was and work toward my own health. Things were going so well I even earned the Employee of the Month Award in July. And things were rolling. I was getting stronger, my endurance was improving, and I felt great.

Unfortunately my GVHD that had all but disappeared with the Pentastatin treatments started to come back. The scarred skin was thickening again, so they started me on Jakafi, the first FDA approved medication specifically for GVHD. I could tell a positive change within a few weeks, and was feeling so good, I started thinking toward the future and what I wanted to do. I got the approval from my doctors to get my MMR immunization which would free me to travel. That was GREAT news!!

This was a really big decision for me because the last time I got a shot, it created a tremendous GVHD response that rocked my world. It took me 2 years to recover from that and I'm still working on what broke. I was thrilled when after 2-3 days I had ZERO symptoms of GVHD and was feeling terrific. It's like my body said, "is that all you got?". So with that behind me, I scheduled the procedure to remove my wisdom teeth. It was something I'd needed to do since before cancer, and now that the chemo and radiation were wreaking havoc on my enamel and gums, it was time to start getting the junk out.

I sailed through that without a hitch, no pain or swelling, and easy recovery. However, when they pulled those teeth, they also took ALL my energy, endurance, strength and drive and replaced it with fatigue and weakness. So this brings me to present time.

I went back to work on a limited basis and the club has been simply terrific and worked with me with amazing grace through this latest setback. So I'm finding purpose again. And seeing more good than bad. I've been able to really be a mom this year and I've loved the time shared with John. I know I'm lucky to have this time with him as a senior in high school, as he'll be going to CSU in the fall. My down time has allowed me to finish this book, and I can't wait to get this into the hands of other patients and caregivers. I want it to be insightful, thoughtful, entertaining, real, and honest.

I have a lot to think about for the future. A lot of opportunities I opened for myself in the past are still there. I'm going to start holding Vision Board classes/retreats at recreation centers, libraries, and hospitals. Some for profit, some not. I taught vision boards to my AVID students and they are very powerful tools for discovering who you are and what you want. I think this would be amazing for cancer patients. Help them find their new normal, really dig into who they are, and give them something to run toward, not run away from. I might get back to my small Christmas Tree business (Tree-t Yourself). I used to make personalized Christmas trees with every theme you can imagine. Sports teams, hobbies (fishing, gardening, books, cooking), favorite color/animal/book, teddy bears, angels, family, and on and on. It was really fun and now with the social media outlet for business, I can imagine it really taking off.

And me. I've lost me. But I'm still in there somewhere. I hate that I can't climb a flight of stairs without having to pause to catch my breath, but that doesn't have to be permanent. Unfortunately the one thing that hospitals don't focus on are the things that are naturally healing processes. It's all about the treatments and the science and the medicines. But there's no integration of cleansing (it's looked down on because it could negatively affect the medication effectiveness), natural remedies like essential oils – even for mood or energy, nutrition, or mental health. You're just thrown out there to find it on your own. But that's an exhausting process and putting the pieces together on your own seems entirely impossible. But I've slowly been gathering the pieces and am putting them in place as I go.

The next leg of this journey must focus on me. I am still working at Lifetime Fitness and surrounded with exceptional people with gigantic hearts who want me to get better. Joe and John are doing the best they can with my daily mood swings and emotions, but I know the more I focus on me, the more "me" will come back. It's a new year which is a great time to start new habits and have an open mind. Not enough of the year has passed to make a judgement if it'll be a good one or bad, but either way, I intend to live the best I can with permission to feel the letdowns and hurdle the bumps as they come.

Who knows… maybe I'll write another book!

CPSIA information can be obtained
at www.ICGtesting.com
Printed in the USA
LVHW07s1327230418
574462LV00001B/1/P